Development and Application of
Herbal Medicine from Marine Origin

Development and Application of Herbal Medicine from Marine Origin

Special Issue Editors

Tsong-Long Hwang
Ping-Jyun Sung
Chih-Chuang Liaw

MDPI • Basel • Beijing • Wuhan • Barcelona • Belgrade

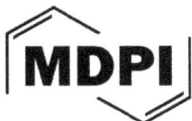

MDPI

Special Issue Editors

Tsong-Long Hwang
Chang Gung University
Taiwan

Ping-Jyun Sung
National Museum of Marine Biology and Aquarium
Taiwan

Chih-Chuang Liaw
National Sun Yat-sen University
Taiwan

Editorial Office
MDPI
St. Alban-Anlage 66
4052 Basel, Switzerland

This is a reprint of articles from the Special Issue published online in the open access journal *Marine Drugs* (ISSN 1660-3397) from 2017 to 2019 (available at: https://www.mdpi.com/journal/marinedrugs/special_issues/Herbal_Medicine_from_Marine)

For citation purposes, cite each article independently as indicated on the article page online and as indicated below:

LastName, A.A.; LastName, B.B.; LastName, C.C. Article Title. *Journal Name* **Year**, *Article Number*, Page Range.

ISBN 978-3-03921-221-7 (Pbk)
ISBN 978-3-03921-222-4 (PDF)

Cover image courtesy of Ping-Jyun Sung.

Contents

About the Special Issue Editors

Tsong-Long Hwang, PhD, is a Professor of the Graduate Institute of Natural Products, Chang Gung University, and a Dean of the College of Human Ecology, Chang Gung University of Science and Technology, Taiwan. He also currently serves as a President of the Society of Chinese Natural Medicine. He received his PhD in Pharmacology at the National Taiwan University in 2000. His research interests include inflammopharmacology, innate immunity, signal transduction, and phytomedicine. His overall goals are to understand the molecular mechanisms in neutrophil activation and to study the pharmacological actions of bioactive compounds in order to develop better therapeutic strategies to treat immune-mediated inflammatory disorders. Dr. Hwang has published more than 300 SCI research articles and has obtained many invention patents.

Ping-Jyun Sung, PhD, obtained his BSc, MSc, and PhD degrees from the National Sun Yat-sen University (NSYSU), where he studied the isolation and structural elucidation of bioactive marine natural products under the guidance of Prof. Sheu from 1989–2000. He undertook a postdoctoral task for Prof. Pettit at the Cancer Research Institute, Arizona State University (ASU-CRI), from 2001–2002, following which he joined the faculties of the National Museum of Marine Biology and Aquarium (NMMBA) and the Graduate Institute of Marine Biology, National Dong Hwa University (NDHU), Taiwan, where he is now a research fellow and Professor, respectively. Dr. Sung's present research interests are related to marine natural products.

Chih-Chuang Liaw, PhD, is a Professor and Chairman of the Department of Marine Biotechnology and Resources, National Sun Yat-Sen University, Taiwan. He received his PhD degree in Natural Products at Kaohsiung Medical University in 2004. His research interests include marine microbial natural products, dereplication, symbiotic microbes, and biofunctional activities. Dr. Liaw has published over 80 SCI research articles.

Preface to "Development and Application of Herbal Medicine from Marine Origin"

Marine herbal medicine generally refers to the use of marine plants as original materials to develop crude drugs, or for other medical purposes. The term 'marine plants' usually denotes macroalgae grown between intertidal and subintertidal zones, including Chlorophyta, Phaeophyta, and Rhodophyta. Considerable progress has been made in the field of biomedical research into marine microalgae and microorganisms in the past decade. As the most important source of fundamental products in the world, marine plants have a very important role in biomedical research. Furthermore, worldwide studies have consistently demonstrated that many crude drugs derived from marine plants contain novel ingredients that may benefit health or can be used in the treatment of diseases; some have been developed into health foods, and some even into drugs. It is expected that there are many substances of marine plant origin that will have medical applications in terms of improving human health and are awaiting discovery.

With the opening of this Special Issue, we aim to draw attention to the scientific research and potential utilization of marine herbal medicines.

Tsong-Long Hwang, Ping-Jyun Sung, Chih-Chuang Liaw
Special Issue Editors

marine drugs

MDPI

Article

Inhibitory Growth of Oral Squamous Cell Carcinoma Cancer via Bacterial Prodigiosin

Ming-Fang Cheng [1,2], Chun-Shu Lin [3], Yu-Hsin Chen [4,5], Ping-Jyun Sung [4,5,6], Shian-Ren Lin [4], Yi-Wen Tong [4] and Ching-Feng Weng [4,5,*]

[1] Department of Pathology, Tri-Service General Hospital, National Defense Medical Center, Taipei 10086, Taiwan; drminfung@gmail.com
[2] Division of Histology and Clinical Pathology, Hualian Army Forces General Hospital, Hualien 97144, Taiwan
[3] Department of Radiation Oncology, Tri-Service General Hospital, National Defense Medical Center, Taipei 10086, Taiwan; Chunshulin@gmail.com
[4] Department of Life Science and Institute of Biotechnology, National Dong Hwa University, Hualien 97401, Taiwan; 810013103@gms.ndhu.edu.tw (Y.-H.C.); pjsung@nmmba.gov.tw (P.-J.S.); d9813003@gms.ndhu.edu.tw (S.-R.L.); mecurry@gmail.com (Y.-W.T.)
[5] Graduate Institute of Marine Biotechnology, National Dong Hwa University, Pingtung 94450, Taiwan
[6] National Museum of Marine Biology and Aquarium, Pingtung 94450, Taiwan
* Correspondence: cfweng@gms.ndhu.edu.tw; Tel.: +886-3-863-3637; Fax: +886-3-863-0255

Received: 11 May 2017; Accepted: 13 July 2017; Published: 15 July 2017

Abstract: Chemotherapy drugs for oral cancers always cause side effects and adverse effects. Currently natural sources and herbs are being searched for treated human oral squamous carcinoma cells (OSCC) in an effort to alleviate the causations of agents in oral cancers chemotherapy. This study investigates the effect of prodigiosin (PG), an alkaloid and natural red pigment as a secondary metabolite of *Serratia marcescens*, to inhibit human oral squamous carcinoma cell growth; thereby, developing a new drug for the treatment of oral cancer. In vitro cultured human OSCC models (OECM1 and SAS cell lines) were used to test the inhibitory growth of PG via cell cytotoxic effects (MTT assay), cell cycle analysis, and Western blotting. PG under various concentrations and time courses were shown to effectively cause cell death and cell-cycle arrest in OECM1 and SAS cells. Additionally, PG induced autophagic cell death in OECM1 and SAS cells by LC3-mediated P62/LC3-I/LC3-II pathway at the in vitro level. These findings elucidate the role of PG, which may target the autophagic cell death pathways as a potential agent in cancer therapeutics.

Keywords: prodigiosin; marine viva; autophage; oral squamous cell carcinoma

---

1. Introduction

Oral cancer is the main cause of cancer death in males in Taiwan and is ranked the fourth leading cause of death overall. Oral cancer mortality and incidence data show that men with oral cancer increases annually. This trend derives from men smoking cigarettes, drinking alcohol, and chewing betel nut. Surprisingly, when a human subject has all three of these habits, the relative risk of oral cancer increases by 122.8 times [1]. Oral squamous cell carcinoma (OSCC) is common in both genders, followed by verrucous carcinoma, undifferentiated carcinoma, and small salivary adenocarcinoma. OSCC is a common type of head and neck cancer [2], excluding oropharynx and hypopharynx. OSCC is locally destructive, may invade the soft tissue and bone, and can be extended to nerves, lymphatic system, and blood vessels. Through these mechanisms, it can spread throughout the body and cause cervical lymph nodes metastasis and distant metastasis [3]. To avoid burdens of the chemotherapy agent in cancer patients, the inductions of cell apoptosis and autophagy are taken firstly into consideration during therapy regimen. This theme is becoming the critical standard for anti-cancer drug discovery.

Autophagy has been shown to be an intracellular degradation process in eukaryotic cells in response to stress, including starvation, clearing damaged proteins and organelles, and promoting cell survival [4,5]. Furthermore, autophagy occurs in multiple processes including nucleation, expansion, and maturation/retrieval to exert the effects of either autophagic cell death or cytoprotection [6]. Currently, two pathways have been investigated to associate with the regulation of autophagy in mammalian cells including the PI3K Class III/Akt/mTOR/p70S6K signaling pathway and the Ras/Raf/MEK/ERK1/2 pathway [7,8]. The ERK1/2 pathway could positively activate autophagy, whereas the Akt/mTOR pathway might suppress autophagy. These signaling pathways could be activated in numerous tumors and are thought to trigger the autophagy and oncogenesis [9]. The stimulation of mTOR protein level is a central regulator of autophagy [10]. Moreover, Akt was associated with cell survival and its expression could down-regulate the LC3-II expression; thereby, suppressing autophagy [11–13]. The amount of LC3-II is demonstrated to correlate well with the amount of autophagosomes [1,14].

Prodigiosin (PG, PubChem CID: 5377753), an alkaloid and natural red pigment, that is a secondary metabolite of *Serratia marcescens*. It is characterized by a common pyrrolyl pyrromethene skeleton [15,16]. Bacterial PGs and their synthetic derivatives have antimicrobial (bactericidal and bacteriostatic) [17–20], antimalarial [17,18,21], and antitumor [17,18,22–24] properties. Additionally, they have been shown to be effective apoptotic agents against various cancer cell lines [25], with multiple cellular targets, including multi-drug resistant cells with little or no toxicity towards normal cell lines, and induce apoptosis in T and B lymphocytes [26,27]. Moreover, PG and its structural analogue (compound R) have induced the expression of p53 target genes accompanied by cell-cycle arrest and apoptosis in p53-deficient cancer cells [28]. PG could be effective as a potential inhibitor compound against COX-2 protein, and can be applied as an anti-inflammatory drug [29]. In melanoma cells, PG activates the mitochondrial apoptotic pathway by disrupting an anti-apoptotic member of the BCL-2 family-MCL-1/BAK complexes by binding to the BH3 domain [30]. Additionally, PG exerts nearly identical cytotoxic effects on the resistant cells in comparison to their parental lines, revealing that this pro-apoptotic agent acts independently on the overexpression of multi-drug resistance transporters-MDR1, BCRP, or MRP [31]. Mechanistically, PG engages the IRE1-JNK and PERK-eIF2α branches of the UPR signaling to up-regulate CHOP, which in turn mediates BCL-2 suppression to induce cell death in multiple human breast carcinoma cell lines [32].

Anti-cancer chemical drugs for oral cancer include 5-FU, cisplatin, paclitaxel, and Ufur. Nonetheless, these chemotherapy drugs always induce side effects, such as nausea, vomiting, loss of appetite, decreased immunity, and adverse effects of oral ulcers. Recently, many natural sources [33–37] and traditional medicinal herbs [38–40] have been studied on OSCC in an effort to mitigate the abovementioned problems, however the solicitation remains incompletely explored. The present study investigated whether PG could have benefits to cause the inhibiting growth of human gingival squamous carcinoma cells (OECM-1) and human tongue cancer (SAS) cell lines by 3-(4,5-Dimethylthiazol-2-yl)-2,5-diphenyltetrazolium bromide (MTT) assay, flow cytometry assay, Western blotting and autophagosome formation assay.

2. Results and Discussion

2.1. Effect of Prodigiosin on the Cell Viability of Oral Cancer Cells

To determine the cytotoxicity of PG in normal cell, normal mouse hepatocyte FL83B cell line was examined. The cell viability of FL83B with various concentration of PG treatment was found no significant cytotoxicity of PG treatment except less cytotoxicity at 25 μM (Figure 1A). In addition, SAS and OECM1 cells were initially treated with 0.1, 0.5, 1.0, and 5.0 μM of PG for 24 h to measure cell viability for the cytotoxic effect of PG. The viable SAS and OECM1 cells were significantly decreased after PG treatment in a dose-dependent manner (Figure 1B,C). The values of IC$_{50}$ on OECM1 and SAS cells were also determined at the concentrations of 1.59 $\pm$ 0.77 and 3.25 $\pm$ 0.49 μM of PG, respectively.

This result indicated that the low concentration of PG elicits the cytotoxicity of OSCC as compared to the untreated cells. Previous reports have demonstrated that PG could cause cell death via apoptotic cell death in several tumors, including human leukemia cells, melanoma, neuroblastoma, colorectal cancer, and breast cancer [32,41,42]. PG and its structural analogue (compound R) are also proven to induce cell-cycle arrest by the expression of p53 target genes in p53-deficient cancer cells [28]. Additionally, as p53 tumor suppressor integrated multiple stress signals, serial anti-proliferative responses would occur to induce apoptosis [43]. In this study, firstly, we presented the inhibitory growth role of PG in human oral squamous cell carcinoma cells in vitro and loss of cell viability was initially found in OECM1 and SAS cells with a dose-dependent fashion after 24 h incubation of PG (Figure 1). Moreover, the IC_{50} of PG on OECM1 and SAS cells were in the low and potential extent.

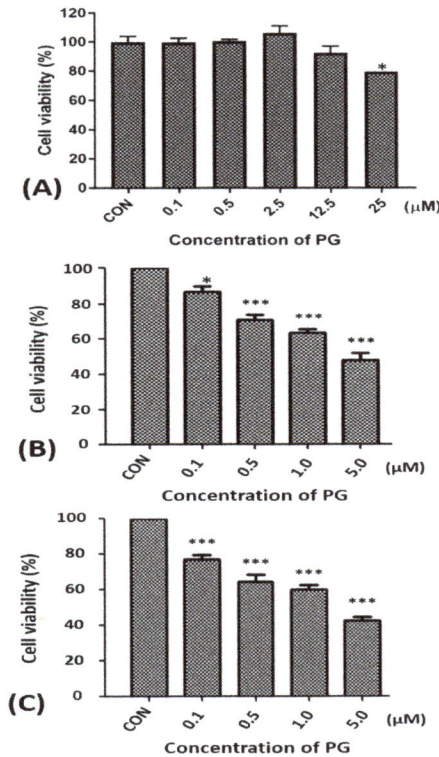

Figure 1. Alterations of the cell viability of FL83B, SAS, and OECM1 cells after prodigiosin treatment. (**A**) FL83B cells were incubated with 0.1 to 25 μM of prodigiosin (PG) for 24 h, (**B**) SAS and (**C**) OECM1 cells were incubated with 0.1, 0.5, 1.0, and 5.0 μM of PG for 24 h, and cell viability was determined by 3-(4,5-Dimethylthiazol-2-yl)-2,5-diphenyltetrazolium bromide (MTT) assay. The data are shown as the mean ± SEM of three independent experiments. * $P < 0.05$; *** $P < 0.001$ when compared with the untreated controls (0 μM).

2.2. Effect of Prodigiosin on the Cell Cycle of Oral Cancer Cells

Obviously, cell cycle of SAS cells after 12 and 24 h of PG treatments showed different pattern. In 12 h treatments of PG, sub-G_1 and S phase of SAS cells were not significantly different and G_0/G_1 phase of SAS cells raised from 40.3 ± 3.3% to 51.4 ± 1.2% ($P < 0.05$). G_2/M phase of SAS cells was decreased from 32.4 ± 2.9% to 27.2 ± 0.7% ($P < 0.05$). In 24 h treatments of PG, S phase of SAS cells was still not significantly different but sub-G_1 and G_0/G_1 phase of SAS cells were elevated from $0.9 \pm 0.3\%$ to $2.5 \pm 0.7\%$ and $42.1 \pm 2.7\%$ to $54.0 \pm 3.7\%$, respectively ($P < 0.05$). G_2/M phase of SAS cells was also decreased from $36.6 \pm 2.1\%$ to $26.3 \pm 3.2\%$ ($P < 0.05$; Table 1).

As SAS cells, sub-G_1 phase of OECM1 cells in 12 h treatments of PG were not significantly different but G_0/G_1 phase of OECM1 cells was significantly increased from $50.9 \pm 1.7\%$ to $63.3 \pm 0.4\%$ ($P < 0.05$). S and G_2/M phase of OECM1 cells were decreased from $16.6 \pm 1.0\%$ to $10.5 \pm 0.2\%$ and $32.1 \pm 0.4\%$ to $25.7 \pm 0.8\%$, respectively ($P < 0.05$). In 24 h treatments of PG, sub-G_1 phase of OECM1 cells was not significantly different but G_2/M phase of OECM1 cells was decreased from $36.9 \pm 3.1\%$ to $18.7 \pm 3.3\%$, respectively ($P < 0.05$). G_0/G_1 and S phase of OECM1 cells were increased from $47.9 \pm 2.3\%$ to $61.8 \pm 0.4\%$ and $14.0 \pm 1.6\%$ to $18.4 \pm 2.6\%$, respectively ($P < 0.05$; Table 2). The above results indicated that PG might inhibit cell growth via arresting cell cycle in G_0/G_1 phase. The protein level of cyclin D1 was analyzed to ensure the hypothesis of cell cycle arrest. Cyclin D1 in two cell lines was significantly decreased after 0.5 and 1.0 μM of PG treatments, which was consistent with the result of cell cycle analysis ($P < 0.05$; Figure 2A,B). These findings indicated that PG could induce cell cycle arrest and delay cell cycle progression, which attributed to inhibitory growth effects of PG in oral cancer cells. In addition, the cell cycle distribution after PG stimulation was observed to arrest in G_0/G_1 phase of SAS cells with various concentrations of PG treatment for 12 h, and in G_0/G_1 phase of OECM1 cells with various concentrations of PG treatment for 12 and 24 h. The findings demonstrated that PG could induce type II program (autophagy) cell death in these cancer cells in a time- and dose-dependent manner. Moreover, there was no significant change of sub-G_1 level in OECM1 and SAS cells after 24 h treatment of PG. We also discovered GFP-LC3 puncta formation in PG-treated OECM1 and SAS cells, which indicated an increase of autophagosome formation in two oral cancer cells (data not shown).

Table 1. Prodigiosin mediated cell cycle distribution in SAS cells.

Cell	Dosage (μM)	Sub G_1 (%)	G_0/G_1 (%)	S (%)	G_2/M (%)
12 h	0	2.2 ± 0.8	40.3 ± 3.3	25.2 ± 4.4	32.4 ± 2.9
	0.1	1.7 ± 0.8	45.3 ± 4.1 *	23.2 ± 0.2	29.9 ± 0.9
	0.5	1.0 ± 0.2	51.2 ± 1.9 *	21.1 ± 2.8	26.6 ± 0.7 *
	1.0	1.4 ± 0.7	51.4 ± 1.2 *	20.0 ± 2.7	27.2 ± 0.2 *
24 h	0	0.9 ± 0.3	42.1 ± 2.7	20.4 ± 2.7	36.6 ± 2.1
	0.1	1.4 ± 0.2	39.7 ± 2.2	25.0 ± 2.0	33.9 ± 3.6
	0.5	1.7 ± 0.3 *	51.7 ± 3.2 *	20.9 ± 0.8	25.7 ± 2.5 *
	1.0	2.5 ± 0.7 *	54.0 ± 3.7 *	17.0 ± 0.7	26.3 ± 3.2 *

SAS cells were treated with 0.1, 0.5, and 1.0 μM of prodigiosin (PG) for 12 and 24 h, respectively, and stained with propidium iodide. The results are shown as the mean ± SEM of three independent experiments. * $P < 0.05$, compared with the untreated control (0 μM).

Table 2. Prodigiosin mediated cell cycle distribution in OECM1 cells.

Cell	Dosage (μM)	Sub G_1 (%)	G_0/G_1 (%)	S (%)	G_2/M (%)
12 h	0	0.5 ± 0.1	50.9 ± 1.7	16.6 ± 1.0	32.1 ± 0.4
	0.1	0.5 ± 0.2	52.3 ± 0.5	17.0 ± 0.5	30.2 ± 2.2
	0.5	0.4 ± 0.1	63.2 ± 0.6 **	12.2 ± 0.2 *	24.1 ± 1.3 *
	1.0	0.4 ± 0.1	63.3 ± 0.4 **	10.5 ± 0.2 *	25.7 ± 0.8 *
24 h	0	1.2 ± 0.2	47.9 ± 2.3	14.0 ± 1.6	36.9 ± 3.1
	0.1	1.1 ± 0.1	50.9 ± 3.8	21.9 ± 2.9 *	26.1 ± 1.6 *
	0.5	1.4 ± 0.1	60.2 ± 2.5 *	19.8 ± 3.1 *	18.7 ± 2.3 **
	1.0	1.2 ± 0.1	61.8 ± 0.4 *	18.4 ± 2.6 *	18.7 ± 3.3 **

OECM1 cells were treated with 0.1, 0.5, and 1.0 μM of prodigiosin (PG) for 12 and 24 h, respectively, and stained with propidium iodide. The results are shown as the mean ± SEM of three independent experiments. * $P < 0.05$ and ** $P < 0.01$, compared with the untreated control (0 μM).

SAS

(A)

OECM1

(B)

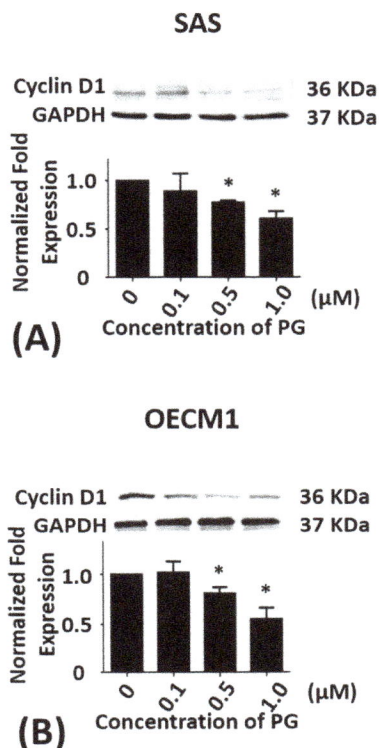

Figure 2. Altered protein levels of cyclin D1 of SAS and OECM1 cells treated with prodigiosin. SAS and OECM1 cells were treated with 0.1, 0.5, and 1.0 μM of prodigiosin (PG) for 24 h and lysed in RIPA buffer for Western blotting. Protein level of cyclin D1 in SAS (**A**) and OECM1 (**B**) cells were shown as the mean ± SEM of three independent experiments. Protein levels were represented as ratio of band intensity to untreated control, which were normalized via internal control GAPDH. * $P < 0.05$ when compared with the untreated control (0 μM).

2.3. Effects of Prodigiosin on AMPKα, PI3K Class III and Akt Protein Levels in Oral Cancer Cells

Cumulative studies have shown that autophagy is mediated by numerous signaling pathway including PI3K/Akt/mTOR [7,8], AMPK/mTOR/Ulk1 [44,45], and Beclin-1 [46]. To evaluate whether PG-induced cell death was related to autophagy, the autophagy-related protein levels of AMPKα, PI3K Class III, Akt, mTOR, Beclin-1, P62, LC3-I, and LC3-II in SAS and OECM1 cells were determined by Western blotting analysis. Compared with the untreated controls, the protein levels of AMPKα in SAS cells exhibited significant differences at 1.0 μM of PG treatment ($P < 0.05$; Figure 3A) while the protein levels of AMPKα in OECM1 cells showed no significant differences in various concentrations of PG treatment (Figure 3B).

When compared with the untreated control, the protein levels of PI3K class III in SAS cells showed no significance (Figure 3C). While the protein levels of PI3K class III in OECM1 cells were markedly down-regulated in 0.5 and 1.0 μM of PG treatments ($P < 0.05$; Figure 3D). The protein level of Akt in SAS and OECM1 cells were evaluated with 0.1, 0.5, and 1.0 μM of PG for 24 h treatments, the results revealed no significant alteration when compared with the untreated controls except significant decrease in 1.0 μM of PG in SAS cells (Figure 3E,F).

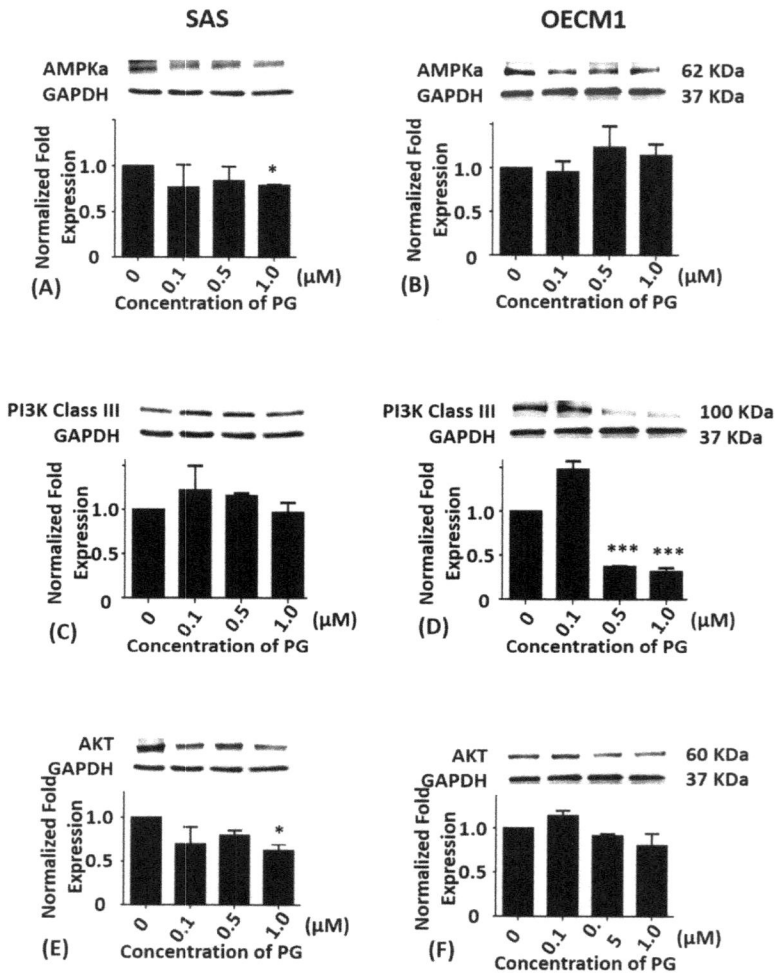

Figure 3. Altered protein levels of AMPKα, PI3K class III, and Akt of SAS and OECM1 cells treated with prodigiosin. SAS and OECM1 cells were treated with 0.1, 0.5, and 1.0 μM of prodigiosin (PG) for 24 h and lysed in RIPA buffer for Western blotting. Protein levels of AMPKα (**A,B**), PI3K class III (**C,D**), and Akt (**E,F**) were shown as the mean ± SEM of three independent experiments. Protein levels were represented as ratio of band intensity to untreated control which were normalized via internal control GAPDH. * $P < 0.05$ and *** $P < 0.001$ when compared with the untreated control (0 μM).

2.4. Effects of Prodigiosin on mTOR and Beclin-1 Protein Levels in Oral Cancer Cells

SAS and OECM1 cells were incubated with 0.1, 0.5, and 1.0 μM of PG treatment for 24 h. As compared with the untreated controls, the protein levels of mTOR in SAS cells were significantly decreased in 1.0 μM of PG treatment ($P < 0.05$; Figure 4A). The protein levels of mTOR in OECM1 cells were also reduced in 0.5 and 1.0 μM of PG treatments ($P < 0.05$; Figure 4B). After treatment with 0.1, 0.5, and 1.0 μM of PG for 24 h, the protein levels of Beclin-1 were significantly decreased in 1.0 μM of PG treatment in SAS and OECM1 cells when compared with the untreated controls ($P < 0.05$; Figure 4C,D).

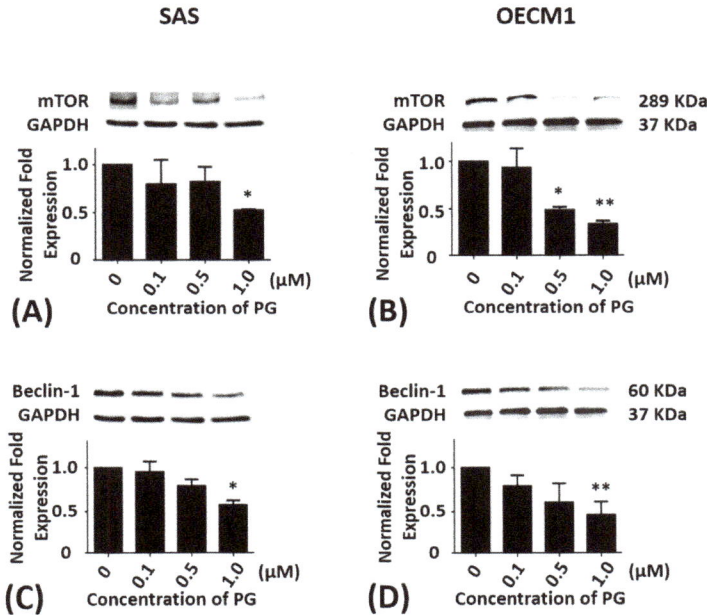

Figure 4. Altered protein levels of mTOR and Beclin-1 of SAS and OECM1 cells treated with prodigiosin. SAS and OECM1 cells were treated with 0.1, 0.5, and 1.0 μM of prodigiosin (PG) for 24 h and lysed in RIPA buffer for Western blotting. Protein levels of mTOR (**A,B**) and Beclin-1 (**C,D**) were shown as the mean ± SEM of three independent experiments. Protein levels were represented as ratio of band intensity to untreated control which were normalized via internal control GAPDH. * $P < 0.05$ and ** $P < 0.01$ when compared with the untreated controls (0 μM).

2.5. Effects of Prodigiosin on P62, LC3-I and LC3-II Protein Levels in Oral Cancer Cells

Additionally, the P62 protein levels in SAS and OECM1 cells were significantly elevated in 1.0 μM of PG treatments as compared with the untreated controls ($P < 0.05$; Figure 5A,B). When compared with the untreated controls, the protein levels of LC3-I in SAS and OECM1 cells were elevated in 1.0 μM of PG treatments ($P < 0.05$; Figure 5C). The protein levels of LC3-I in OECM1 showed a significant increase in various concentrations of PG for 24 h treatment ($P < 0.05$; Figure 5D). The protein levels of LC3-II were markedly up-regulated in SAS cells with various concentrations of PG treatment for 24 h as compared with the untreated controls ($P < 0.05$; Figure 5E). While the protein levels of LC3-II also revealed a large increase in OECM1 cells with 0.5 and 1.0 μM of PG treatment for 24 h as compared with the untreated controls ($P < 0.05$; Figure 5F). These Western-blotting findings showed that autophagic cell death could be induced by PG treatment in oral cancer cells, which might occur through different signal pathways. Remarkably, the increase of P62, LC3-I, and LC3-II levels in the present study is associated with numerous investigations. Two carbazole alkaloids derived from *Murraya koenigii* (L.) Sprengel (Rutaceae) leaves, mahanine and isomahanine, resulted in increased accumulation of p62/sequestosome1 (p62/SQSTM1), with coordinated expression of LC3-II and cleaved caspase-3, suggesting inhibition of autophagic flux associated with carbazole alkaloid-induced apoptosis in the OSCC cell line CLS-354 [40]. Protein levels of LC3-II and p62 in human breast cancer cell lines MCF-7 and MDA-MB-231 are induced by ramalin that derived from the Antarctic lichen *Ramalina terebrata* [47]. One more recent report has demonstrated the autophagic cell death of HepG$_2$ by dehydroepiandrosterone treatment and also via an increase of JNK-mediated P62 expression [48]. Nutrient depletion has augmented OSCC cell autophagy via increase of p62, LC3-II/LC3-I ratio, and GFP-LC3 levels in time-course patterns from 6 to 48 h when the inhibition of autophagy caused apoptosis in OSCC cells [49]. In study of anticancer effect of ursolic acid in apoptosis-resistant colorectal cancer, JNK signaling pathway has been triggered and further activated P62 expression [50]. Resveratrol can enhance autophagy via increase of JNK-mediated P62 expression and AMPK activation in chronic myelogenous leukemia cells [51,52]. Conversely, isomahanine, a carbazole alkaloid, obviously induces autophagic flux as shown by an increase in punctate GFP-LC3 and the LC3-II/LC3-I ratio with a concomitant p62 level decrease in multidrug-resistant human oral squamous cell carcinoma cells [53]. Treatment with grape seed extract and resveratrol in 4-nitroquinoline-1-oxide (4NQO)-induced tongue tumorigenesis of C57BL/6 mice, that decrease of autophagy flux marker p62 is observed [54]. Human lung cancer tissues that experienced chemotherapy shows an increase of LC3-I to LC3-II conversion and decrease of p62/sequestosome1 as compared with chemo-naïve cancer tissue as well as A549 cell [55]. Sunitinib, an oral multitargeted receptor tyrosine kinase inhibitor with antiangiogenic and antitumor activity that mainly targets vascular endothelial growth factor receptors, significantly increases the levels of LC3-II, concomitant with a decrease of p62 in rat pheochromocytoma PC12 cells [56]. Interestingly, the signaling of P62 seems to be a biphasic response for the induction of autophagy.

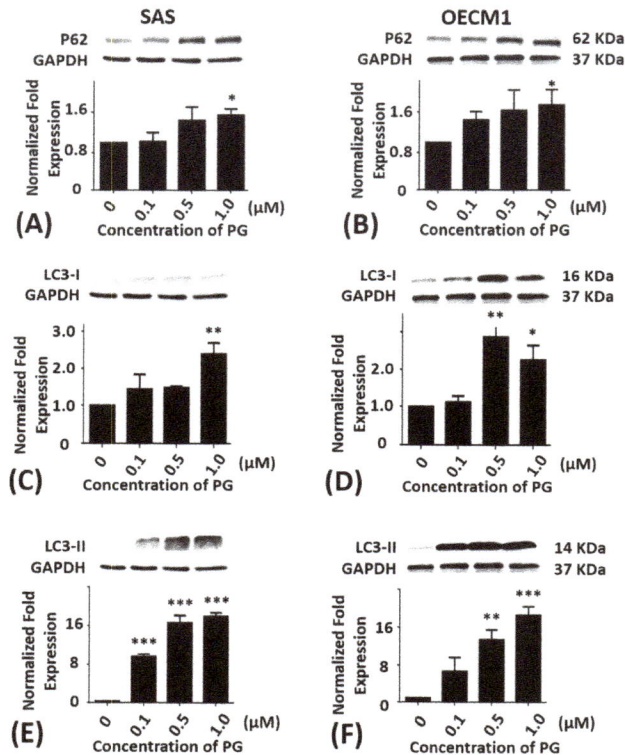

Figure 5. Altered protein levels of P62, LC3-I, and LC3-II of SAS and OECM1 cells treated with prodigiosin. SAS and OECM1 cells were treated with 0.1, 0.5, and 1.0 µM of prodigiosin (PG) for 24 h and lysed in RIPA buffer for Western blotting. Protein levels of P62 (**A**,**B**), LC3-I (**C**,**D**), and LC3-II (**E**,**F**) were shown as the mean ± SEM of three independent experiments. Protein levels were represented as ratio of band intensity to untreated control which were normalized via internal control GAPDH. * $P < 0.05$, ** $P < 0.01$, and *** $P < 0.001$ when compared with the untreated controls (0 µM).

2.6. Phosphorylated Protein Levels of mTOR, Akt, and Ribosomal Protein S6 after PG Treatment

Previous studies have been shown that Akt and mTOR phosphorylation would be reduced while autophagy activation. Moreover, mTOR dephosphorylation reduced downstream protein p70S6K activation and finally inhibited ribosomal protein S6 (rpS6) phosphorylation [57–59]. Consequently, mTOR, Akt and rpS6 phosphorylation could be a marker of autophagy activation. After treatment of 1 µM PG, mTOR, Akt, and rpS6 phosphorylation in both SAS and OECM1 cells were significantly decreased (Figure 6). According to these results, PG could not only reduce mTOR and Akt protein expression, but also inhibit the phosphorylations of mTOR and Akt.

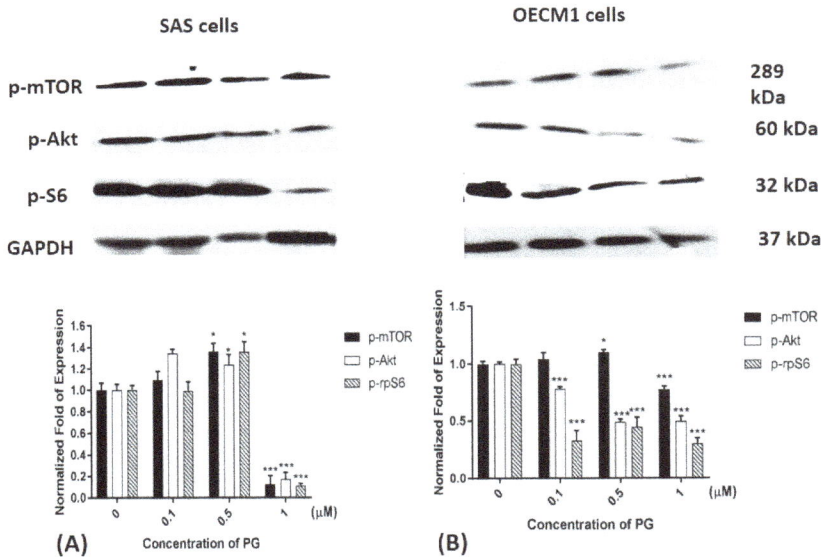

Figure 6. Altered protein levels of p-mTOR, p-Akt, and p-rpS6 of (**A**) SAS and (**B**) OECM1 cells treated with prodigiosin. SAS and OECM1 cells were treated with 0.1, 0.5, and 1.0 µM of prodigiosin (PG) for 24 h and lysed in RIPA buffer for Western blotting. Protein levels of p-mTOR, p-Akt, and p-rpS6 were shown as the mean ± SEM of three independent experiments. Protein levels were represented as ratio of band intensity to untreated control which were normalized via internal control GAPDH. * $P < 0.05$ and *** $P < 0.001$ when compared with the untreated controls (0 µM).

2.7. Effect of Prodigiosin on Autophagosome Formation in Oral Cancer Cells

For evaluating whether autophagy appeared in oral cancer cells after PG treatment, the expressions of LC3-II in autophagosome in SAS and OECM1 cells were further observed via immunofluorescence. During the cascade of autophagy signal pathways, LC3-II can anchor on the autophagosome, and its amount is correlated well with the numbers of autophagosomes [8,14]. Two oral cancer cells were incubated with 0.4 µM PG and 0.4 µM PG plus 5 mM of autophagic inhibitor 3-methyladenine (3MA) for 24 h when compared with the untreated control cells. The results illustrated that increased LC3 puncta cells were significantly increased by presenting numerous autophagosomes in SAS and OECM-1 treated with PG and decreased by the application of 3MA. Figure 7A,B showed the quantitative representations of autophagosome formation in SAS and OECM1 cells ($P < 0.05$). Furthermore, in order to prove PG-induced OSCC cells death was caused by autophagy, cell viability of two OSCC cells were tested after PG treatment with or without 1 mM and 5 mM of 3MA. The data illustrated that cell viability of PG combined with 1 mM 3MA in two cell lines were significantly higher than that of PG alone. However, cell viability of PG combined with 5 mM 3MA was significantly lower than that of PG alone. Meanwhile, 1 and 5 mM of 3MA could increase two cell lines growth (Figure 7C). Previous study has been demonstrated biphasic function of 3MA in cell autophagy. In nutrient-rich environment, 3MA would promote the autophagy [60], which might explain the decrease of cell viability after treatment of 5 mM 3MA plus PG. Take all above results together, autophagy indeed occurred in oral cancer cells in the induction of PG.

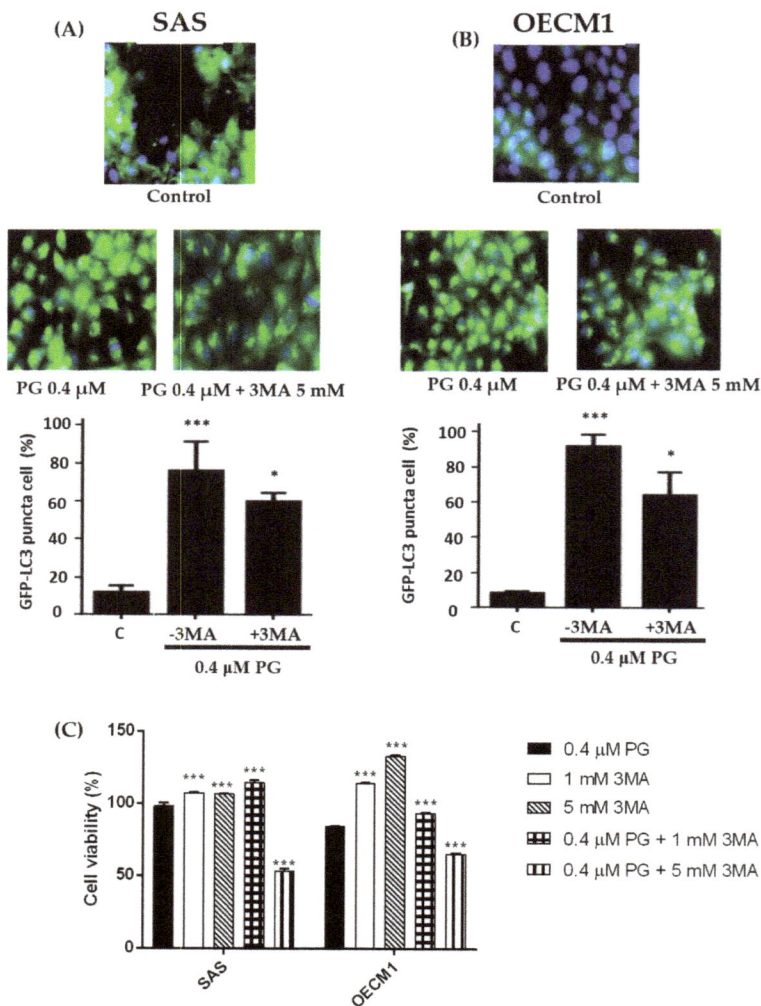

Figure 7. Alterations of autophosome formation of (**A**) SAS and (**B**) OECM1 cells treated with prodigiosin. SAS and OECM1 cells were treated with prodigiosin (PG; 0.1, 0.4, and 1.0 μM) and PG + 3MA (0.4 μM of PG and plus 5 mM of 3MA) for 24 h, followed by staining the autophagosome by LC3 antibody (green) and nucleus by DAPI (blue). The LC3 puncta cells of SAS and OECM1 were observed using fluorescence microscopy and counted the percentage of LC3 positive cell. (**C**) Cytotoxicity of treatment with 0.4 μM of PG + 3MA (1 and 5 mM) in two cell lines was observed by MTT assay. The results were shown as the mean ± SEM of three independent experiments. * $P < 0.05$ and *** $P < 0.001$ when compared with the untreated controls (0 μM).

PG can down-regulate RAD51 expression, and trigger phosphorylation of JNK and p38 MAPK in many human breast carcinoma cell lines, which implicates the cytotoxicity of PG in this cancer [32]. The structural modification of the C-ring of prodigiosenes results in an anti-cancer activity of human K562 chronic myelogenous leukemia cells in both in vitro and in vivo assays [42]. From these data, PGs are thought to play critical roles in cancer therapy via inducing cell death [61]. Recently, PG can induce apoptosis in various cancer cells with low toxicity on normal cells, and PG-induced apoptosis may ascribe to Bcl-2 and survivin inhibition in colorectal cancer (HT-29) cells [62]. In addition, autophagy has been found in squamous cell carcinoma of the head and neck [63]. Increased protein levels of P62 and LC3-II in OSCC tissues have also been reported to correlate with survival, poor prognosis, and advanced stage cancer [64]. In this study, Western blot analyses showed that PG-induced autophagy in OECM1 cells by down-regulation of mTOR, PI3 kinase Class III, and Beclin-1 protein levels while by up-regulation of P62 and LC3 proteins. In SAS cells, PG-induced autophagy was associated with the involvement of decreased signals of mTOR, Akt, and Beclin-1 proteins while increase of P62 and LC3 proteins. Decreased protein level of cyclin D1 after 24 h treatment with 0.5 and 1.0 μM PG was observed in SAS and OECM1 cells (Figure 2), indicating G_0/G_1 checkpoint arrest. Furthermore, marked up-regulation of LC3-I and LC3-II protein levels was exhibited in OSCC cells, and a significant increase was found by presenting numerous autophagosomes in these cancer cells (Figure 7). Thereby, our findings provide the first evidence of increased autophagic signals were involved cell death by PG treatment in OECM1 and SAS cells. These results are consistent with previous findings for cell death of PG induction in melanoma cells of previous report. PG can be a specific mTOR inhibitor in melanoma cells, which might induce a loss of Akt phosphorylation, prevent its activation, and identify a possible new therapeutic option for this cancer [41]. Moreover, Akt is associated with cell survival and its expression could down-regulate the LC3-II expression; thereby, suppressing autophagy [11–13]. The PI3K Class III can be triggered through insulin and insulin-like receptors, for reduction of its signal to Akt; therefore, stimulating the protein level of mTOR, which is a central regulator of autophagy. Subsequently, the activation of mTOR would further suppress the autophagy pathway and induce protein synthesis. In fact, when mTOR is suppressed, autophagy is conversely induced. Autophagy is also promoted by AMP activated protein kinase (AMPK), which is a key energy sensor to maintain energy homeostasis [10].

3. Materials and Methods

3.1. Preparations of Prodigiosin

Vibrio sp. C1-TDSG02-1 was isolated from the sea sediment of Siaogang Harbor at a water depth of 17 m in eastern and southern Taiwan. The strain C1-TDSG02-1 was 99.0% identical with Vibrio sp. BL-182 (Genbank accession no. AY663829.1) based on 16S rDNA gene sequence. Vibrio sp. C1-TDSG02-1 was cultured in 1.4% soybean flour with 80% sterilized seawater at 25 °C, 5 Lpm (L/min), and pH 7.0–7.5 for 48 h. Extraction of the culture broth (8.0 L) with ethyl acetate (EtOAc, 4 × 8.0 L) yielded 45.7 g of crude extract. The EtOAc layer was separated on silica gel followed by elution chromatography with mixed n-hexane/EtOAc (stepwise, pure n-hexane, pure EtOAc) to yield 16 sub-fractions. Fraction 6 was chromatographed on silica and eluted using a mixture of n-hexane/acetone (stepwise, 10:1, pure acetone) to afford 11 sub-fractions. Sub-fraction 6-5 was chromatographed on silica and eluted using a mixture of n-hexane/acetone (4:1) to afford prodigiosin (PG, 1.94 g). The purity of purified PG is 95% confirmed by NMR. Prodigiosin ($C_{20}H_{25}N_3O$; mol. wt.: 323.432 g/mole) was isolated as a red powder that gave an $[M + H]^+$ ion peak at 324 m/z in the ESI/MS. One liter of culture can obtain approximately 1.398 g of PG.

3.2. Cell Cultures

Two human oral squamous carcinoma cell lines (SAS and OECM1) were obtained from Dr. Ta-Chun Yuan of Department of Life Science and Institute of Biotechnology (National Dong-Hwa

University, Hualien, Taiwan). SAS were cultured in Dulbecco's modified Eagle medium (DMEM, Thermo-Fisher, Waltham, MA, USA) supplemented with 5% fetal bovine serum (FBS, Thermo-Fisher), and 1% penicillin/streptomycin (PS, Thermo-Fisher). OECM1 were cultured in Roswell Park Memorial Institute medium 1640 (RPMI 1640) supplemented with 5% FBS and 1% PS. Two cell lines were cultured in CO_2 incubator (Thermo-Fisher) and the culture condition was set up as 37 °C, 5% CO_2. The medium was changed every 2 days, and the cells were detached by 0.25% trypsin/EDTA (Thermo-Fisher) for passage as reached 80–90% confluence. All experiments were obtained within 20 passages concerning uniformity and reproducibility. FL83B (mouse hepatocyte, ATCC CRL-2390) cells were maintained in Kaighn's Modification of Ham's F-12 Medium (F12K, Thermo-Fisher) supplemented with 10% FBS and 1% PS, and incubated at 37 °C with 5% CO_2.

3.3. Cytotoxicity Assay

Cytotoxicity was measured by MTT assay. 7×10^3 cells per well of SAS/OECM1 were seeded in 96-well plates and incubated at 37 °C, 5% CO_2 overnight. Then, the cells were treated with various concentrations of PG (0.1, 0.5, 1.0, and 5.0 µM) for 24 h. After treatment, 20 µL per well of 50 mg/mL MTT (Thermo-Fisher) solution was added and incubated at 37 °C for 3 h. As incubation finished, all liquid in wells were replaced to dimethyl sulfoxide and the absorbance at 570 nm was measured by EnSpire Alpha plate reader (Perkin Elmer, Waltham, MA, USA). The absorbance at 570 nm was positively correlated to the number of viable cells so the cell viability was represented as the percentage of absorbance at 570 nm between treated and untreated cells.

3.4. Cell Cycle Analysis

A total of 7×10^4 cells of SAS/OECM1 were seeded in 12-well plates and incubated at 37 °C, 5% CO_2 overnight. Then, cells were incubated with 0.1, 0.5, and 1.0 µM of PG for 12 and 24 h. Next, cells were harvested by 0.25% trypsin/EDTA and fixed with 70% ethanol at −20 °C at least 1 h. The fixed cells were washed in cold phosphate buffer saline (PBS) twice, stained with 1 mL staining solution (20 µg/mL of propidium iodide (PI), 0.1% Triton X-100, 0.2 mg/mL RNase) at 37 °C for 30 min, and emission density at 617 nm was analyzed within 10^4 cells for each treatment by Cytomics™ FC500 flow cytometer (Beckman Coulter, Brea, CA, USA).

3.5. Western Blotting

A total of 7×10^4 of OECM1 and SAS cell lines were seeded in 12-well plates and cells reached 80% confluence at 37 °C and 5% CO_2. OECM1 and SAS cells were treated with 0.1, 0.5, and 1.0 µM of PG for 24 h. Then, media in wells were removed and washed twice with PBS. Cells in wells were homogenized using RIPA buffer and harvested into a 1.5 mL Eppendorf. The cell lysates were centrifuged at 12,000× *g* at 4 °C for 30 min, and the supernatant was kept at −20 °C until assayed. Interested proteins were separated using sodium dodecyl sulfate polyacrylamide gel electrophoresis and subsequently transferred to PVDF membrane (Millipore, Billerica, MA, USA). The membrane was blocked with 5% non-fat milk or 5% bovine serum albumin (for phosphorylated protein) in TBST saline (20 mM Tris-HCl, pH 7.4, 137 mM NaCl, and 0.05% Tween-20) at room temperature for 1 h, followed by incubation with an appropriate primary antibody at 4 °C overnight. The membrane was washed by TBST saline twice and then incubated with peroxidase conjugated secondary antibody for 1 h. Finally, the membrane was rinsed with ECL reagent (Amershan Bioscience, Little Chalfont, UK) for 1 min and chemiluminescence was collected with a LAS-3000 imager (Fujifilm, Tokyo, Japan). GAPDH was taken as an internal control for normalization. Table 3 shows primary and secondary antibodies used in this study.

Table 3. Primary and second antibodies used in the study.

Antibody	MW(kDa)	Dilution	Sources
mTOR	289	1:1000	Cell Signalling
p-mTOR (Ser2448)	289	1:200	Santa Cruz
PI3K class III	100	1:1000	Cell Signalling
AMPKα	62	1:1000	Cell Signalling
P62	62	1:1000	Cell Signalling
Akt	60	1:1000	Cell Signalling
P-Akt (Ser473)	60	1:200	Santa Cruz
Beclin-1	60	1:1000	Cell Signalling
Cyclin D1	34	1:1000	Cell Signalling
p-Ribosomal protein S6 (Ser235/236)	32	1:200	Santa Cruz
LC3-I	16	1:1000	Cell Signalling
LC3-II	14	1:1000	Cell Signalling
GADPH	37	1:10,000	Cell Signalling
anti-Rabbit (IgG)	-	1:5000	GeneTex
anti-Mouse (IgG)	-	1:10,000	GE

3.6. Autophagosome Formation Analysis

OECM1 and SAS cells were plated into 96-well plates at a cell density of 5×10^3/well. The cells were incubated at 37 °C and 5% CO_2. OECM1 and SAS cells were incubated in 0.4 µM of PG and 0.4 µM of PG plus 5 mM of 3-methyladenine (3MA) for 24 h. Then, cells were fixed with 3.7% formaldehyde/PBS and stained by the Alexa Fluor 488-conjugated anti-LC3-II rabbit antibody (Thermo-Fisher). Images were captured by a Typhoon™ FLA 9000 Biomolecular Imager (GE Healthcare, Little Chalfont, UK). The fluorescence focus units were quantified in each well.

3.7. Statistical Analysis

Data were expressed as mean ± SEM of at least three independent experiments. The results were analyzed by one-way analysis of variance (ANOVA) followed by a Tukey's test. Significant differences ($P < 0.05$) between the means of control and treatment were analyzed. All statistical procedures were performed with GraphPad Prism Ver 5.0 software (GraphPad Software, La Jolla, San Diego, CA, USA).

4. Conclusions

The autophagic mechanism of PG against oral cancer cells was proposed (Figure 8). PG might inhibit cell growth via suppressing the cyclin D1 to cause the arresting cell cycle in G_0/G_1 phase. Furthermore, PG could mediate AMPKα, PI3K class III/Akt signal pathway and directly or indirectly exerts the inhibition of mTOR and Beclin-1 and the induction of p62/LC3 resulting in cell autophagy. In the present study revealed that PG could induce autophagic cell death in human oral cancer cells by LC3-mediated P62/LC3-I/LC3-II pathway in vitro. Our findings elucidated the inhibitory role of PG in this OSCC cancer, which may target the autophagic pathways as a potential agent in cancer therapeutics. Further work in studying anticancer activity of PG should focus on the in vivo test of PG. In a lung cancer xenograft model in vivo studies have demonstrated cancer growth inhibition of tumor growth via cell apoptosis and invasion. Moreover, PG has inhibited RhoA and MMP-2 protein expression in lung cancer 95-D cell line resulting in invasion inhibition [65]. In addition, the activation of p73 and c-Jun-mediated ΔNp73 signaling pathway by PG induced, which can restore p53 tumor suppressor activity in colon cancer [28,66]. In breast cancer, PG could downregulate the Wnt/β-catenin signaling pathway, resulting in the triggered apoptosis process [67]. Based on the present study, this is the first evident that (1) autophagy-induced activity of PG; and (2) growth inhibiting activity of PG in OSCC. This study has confirmed that PG might have a chemotherapeutic potential and promise in treating oral squamous cell carcinoma.

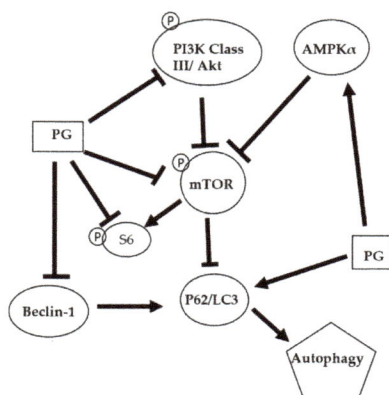

Figure 8. The proposed autophagic mechanism of prodigiosin against oral cancer cells. AMP-activated protein kinase alpha (AMPKα); Mammalian target of rapamycin (mTOR); Microtubule-associated protein 1A/1B-light chain 3 (LC3); Nucleoporin 62 (P62); Phosphoinositide 3-kinase (PI3K); Prodigiosin (PG); Protein kinase B (Akt); and Ribosomal protein S6 (S6)

Acknowledgments: This work was supported by grants from the National Science Council (Ministry of Science and Technology) [Grant 102-2320-B-259-001-3].

Author Contributions: Ming-Fang Cheng, Ping-Jyun Sung and Ching-Feng Weng conceived and designed the experiments. Ming-Fang Cheng, Yi-Wen Tong, Yu-Hsin Chen and Shian-Ren Lin executed the experiments, acquisition and analysis of data. Ming-Fang Cheng, Chun-Shu Lin and Ching-Feng Weng wrote the paper.

Conflicts of Interest: The authors declare no conflicts of interest.

1. Marques, L.A.; Eluf-Neto, J.; Figueiredo, R.A.; Gois-Filho, J.F.; Kowalski, L.P.; Carvalho, M.B.; Abrahao, M.; Wunsch-Filho, V. Oral health, hygiene practices and oral cancer. *Rev. Saude Publica* **2008**, *42*, 471–479. [CrossRef]
2. Sciubba, J.J. Oral cancer. The importance of early diagnosis and treatment. *Am. J. Clin. Dermatol.* **2001**, *2*, 239–251. [CrossRef] [PubMed]
3. Olsen, S.M.; Moore, E.J.; Koch, C.A.; Kasperbauer, J.L.; Olsen, K.D. Oral cavity and oropharynx squamous cell carcinoma with metastasis to the parotid lymph nodes. *Oral Oncol.* **2011**, *47*, 142–144. [CrossRef] [PubMed]
4. Singletary, K.; Milner, J. Diet, autophagy, and cancer: A review. *Cancer Epidemiol. Biomark. Prev.* **2008**, *17*, 1596–1610. [CrossRef] [PubMed]
5. Wu, J.J.; Quijano, C.; Chen, E.; Liu, H.; Cao, L.; Fergusson, M.M.; Rovira, I.I.; Gutkind, S.; Daniels, M.P.; Komatsu, M.; et al. Mitochondrial dysfunction and oxidative stress mediate the physiological impairment induced by the disruption of autophagy. *Aging* **2009**, *1*, 425–437. [CrossRef] [PubMed]
6. Luo, G.X.; Cai, J.; Lin, J.Z.; Luo, W.S.; Luo, H.S.; Jiang, Y.Y.; Zhang, Y. Autophagy inhibition promotes gambogic acid-induced suppression of growth and apoptosis in glioblastoma cells. *Asian Pac. J. Cancer Prev.* **2012**, *13*, 6211–6216. [CrossRef] [PubMed]
7. Shinojima, N.; Yokoyama, T.; Kondo, Y.; Kondo, S. Roles of the akt/mtor/p70s6k and erk1/2 signaling pathways in curcumin-induced autophagy. *Autophagy* **2007**, *3*, 635–637. [CrossRef] [PubMed]
8. Han, H.Y.; Kim, H.; Jeong, S.H.; Lim, D.S.; Ryu, M.H. Sulfasalazine induces autophagic cell death in oral cancer cells via akt and erk pathways. *Asian Pac. J. Cancer Prev.* **2014**, *15*, 6939–6944. [CrossRef] [PubMed]
9. Ellington, A.A.; Berhow, M.A.; Singletary, K.W. Inhibition of akt signaling and enhanced erk1/2 activity are involved in induction of macroautophagy by triterpenoid b-group soyasaponins in colon cancer cells. *Carcinogenesis* **2006**, *27*, 298–306. [CrossRef] [PubMed]
10. Yao, F.; Lv, Y.C.; Zhang, M.; Xie, W.; Tan, Y.L.; Gong, D.; Cheng, H.P.; Liu, D.; Li, L.; Liu, X.Y.; et al. Apelin-13 impedes foam cell formation by activating class iii pi3k/beclin-1-mediated autophagic pathway. *Biochem. Biophys. Res. Commun.* **2015**, *466*, 637–643. [CrossRef] [PubMed]

11. Sarbassov, D.D.; Guertin, D.A.; Ali, S.M.; Sabatini, D.M. Phosphorylation and regulation of akt/pkb by the rictor-mtor complex. *Science* **2005**, *307*, 1098–1101. [CrossRef] [PubMed]

12. Degtyarev, M.; De Maziere, A.; Orr, C.; Lin, J.; Lee, B.B.; Tien, J.Y.; Prior, W.W.; van Dijk, S.; Wu, H.; Gray, D.C.; et al. Akt inhibition promotes autophagy and sensitizes pten-null tumors to lysosomotropic agents. *J. Cell Biol.* **2008**, *183*, 101–116. [CrossRef] [PubMed]

13. Roy, B.; Pattanaik, A.K.; Das, J.; Bhutia, S.K.; Behera, B.; Singh, P.; Maiti, T.K. Role of pi3k/akt/mtor and mek/erk pathway in concanavalin a induced autophagy in hela cells. *Chem. Biol. Interact.* **2014**, *210*, 96–102. [CrossRef] [PubMed]

14. Song, L.; Ma, L.; Chen, G.; Huang, Y.; Sun, X.; Jiang, C.; Liu, H. Autophagy inhibitor 3-methyladenine enhances the sensitivity of nasopharyngeal carcinoma cells to chemotherapy and radiotherapy. *Zhong Nan Da Xue Xue Bao Yi Xue Ban* **2016**, *41*, 9–18. [PubMed]

15. Chang, C.C.; Chen, W.C.; Ho, T.F.; Wu, H.S.; Wei, Y.H. Development of natural anti-tumor drugs by microorganisms. *J. Biosci. Bioeng.* **2011**, *111*, 501–511. [CrossRef] [PubMed]

16. Marchal, E.; Smithen, D.A.; Uddin, M.I.; Robertson, A.W.; Jakeman, D.L.; Mollard, V.; Goodman, C.D.; MacDougall, K.S.; McFarland, S.A.; McFadden, G.I.; et al. Synthesis and antimalarial activity of prodigiosenes. *Org. Biomol. Chem.* **2014**, *12*, 4132–4142. [CrossRef] [PubMed]

17. Lapenda, J.C.; Silva, P.A.; Vicalvi, M.C.; Sena, K.X.; Nascimento, S.C. Antimicrobial activity of prodigiosin isolated from serratia marcescens ufpeda 398. *World J. Microbiol. Biotechnol.* **2015**, *31*, 399–406. [CrossRef] [PubMed]

18. Wang, Y.; Nakajima, A.; Hosokawa, K.; Soliev, A.B.; Osaka, I.; Arakawa, R.; Enomoto, K. Cytotoxic prodigiosin family pigments from *pseudoalteromonas sp.* 1020r isolated from the pacific coast of Japan. *Biosci. Biotechnol. Biochem.* **2012**, *76*, 1229–1232. [CrossRef] [PubMed]

19. Kimyon, O.; Das, T.; Ibugo, A.I.; Kutty, S.K.; Ho, K.K.; Tebben, J.; Kumar, N.; Manefield, M. Serratia secondary metabolite prodigiosin inhibits pseudomonas aeruginosa biofilm development by producing reactive oxygen species that damage biological molecules. *Front. Microbiol.* **2016**, *7*, 972–987. [CrossRef] [PubMed]

20. Song, Y.; Liu, G.; Li, J.; Huang, H.; Zhang, X.; Zhang, H.; Ju, J. Cytotoxic and antibacterial angucycline- and prodigiosin-analogues from the deep-sea derived *streptomyces sp.* Scsio 11594. *Mar. Drugs* **2015**, *13*, 1304–1316. [CrossRef] [PubMed]

21. Kancharla, P.; Lu, W.; Salem, S.M.; Kelly, J.X.; Reynolds, K.A. Stereospecific synthesis of 23-hydroxyundecylprodiginines and analogues and conversion to antimalarial premarineosins via a rieske oxygenase catalyzed bicyclization. *J. Org. Chem.* **2014**, *79*, 11674–11689. [CrossRef] [PubMed]

22. Perez-Tomas, R.; Vinas, M. New insights on the antitumoral properties of prodiginines. *Curr. Med. Chem.* **2010**, *17*, 2222–2231. [CrossRef] [PubMed]

23. Sam, S.; Sam, M.R.; Esmaeillou, M.; Safaralizadeh, R. Effective targeting survivin, caspase-3 and microrna-16–1 expression by methyl-3-pentyl-6-methoxyprodigiosene triggers apoptosis in colorectal cancer stem-like cells. *Pathol. Oncol. Res.* **2016**, *22*, 715–723. [CrossRef] [PubMed]

24. Yu, C.J.; Ou, J.H.; Wang, M.L.; Jialielihan, N.; Liu, Y.H. Elevated survivin mediated multidrug resistance and reduced apoptosis in breast cancer stem cells. *J. BUON* **2015**, *20*, 1287–1294. [PubMed]

25. Papireddy, K.; Smilkstein, M.; Kelly, J.X.; Shweta; Salem, S.M.; Alhamadsheh, M.; Haynes, S.W.; Challis, G.L.; Reynolds, K.A. Antimalarial activity of natural and synthetic prodiginines. *J. Med. Chem.* **2011**, *54*, 5296–5306. [CrossRef] [PubMed]

26. Chang, C.C.; Wang, Y.H.; Chern, C.M.; Liou, K.T.; Hou, Y.C.; Peng, Y.T.; Shen, Y.C. Prodigiosin inhibits gp91(phox) and inos expression to protect mice against the oxidative/nitrosative brain injury induced by hypoxia-ischemia. *Toxicol. Appl. Pharmacol.* **2011**, *257*, 137–147. [CrossRef] [PubMed]

27. Dalili, D.; Fouladdel, S.; Rastkari, N.; Samadi, N.; Ahmadkhaniha, R.; Ardavan, A.; Azizi, E. Prodigiosin, the red pigment of *serratia marcescens*, shows cytotoxic effects and apoptosis induction in ht-29 and t47d cancer cell lines. *Nat. Prod. Res.* **2012**, *26*, 2078–2083. [PubMed]

28. Hong, B.; Prabhu, V.V.; Zhang, S.; van den Heuvel, A.P.; Dicker, D.T.; Kopelovich, L.; El-Deiry, W.S. Prodigiosin rescues deficient p53 signaling and antitumor effects via upregulating p73 and disrupting its interaction with mutant p53. *Cancer Res.* **2014**, *74*, 1153–1165. [CrossRef] [PubMed]

29. Krishna, P.S.; Vani, K.; Prasad, M.R.; Samatha, B.; Bindu, N.S.; Charya, M.A.; Reddy Shetty, P. In silico molecular docking analysis of prodigiosin and cycloprodigiosin as cox-2 inhibitors. *Springerplus* **2013**, *2*, 172–178. [CrossRef] [PubMed]

30. Hosseini, A.; Espona-Fiedler, M.; Soto-Cerrato, V.; Quesada, R.; Perez-Tomas, R.; Guallar, V. Molecular interactions of prodiginines with the bh3 domain of anti-apoptotic bcl-2 family members. *PLoS ONE* **2013**, *8*, e57562. [CrossRef] [PubMed]

31. Elahian, F.; Moghimi, B.; Dinmohammadi, F.; Ghamghami, M.; Hamidi, M.; Mirzaei, S.A. The anticancer agent prodigiosin is not a multidrug resistance protein substrate. *DNA Cell Biol.* **2013**, *32*, 90–97. [CrossRef] [PubMed]

32. Pan, M.Y.; Shen, Y.C.; Lu, C.H.; Yang, S.Y.; Ho, T.F.; Peng, Y.T.; Chang, C.C. Prodigiosin activates endoplasmic reticulum stress cell death pathway in human breast carcinoma cell lines. *Toxicol. Appl. Pharmacol.* **2012**, *265*, 325–334. [CrossRef] [PubMed]

33. Chang, Y.T.; Huang, C.Y.; Li, K.T.; Li, R.N.; Liaw, C.C.; Wu, S.H.; Liu, J.R.; Sheu, J.H.; Chang, H.W. Sinuleptolide inhibits proliferation of oral cancer ca9–22 cells involving apoptosis, oxidative stress, and DNA damage. *Arch. Oral Biol.* **2016**, *66*, 147–154. [CrossRef] [PubMed]

34. Dai, W.; Sun, C.; Huang, S.; Zhou, Q. Carvacrol suppresses proliferation and invasion in human oral squamous cell carcinoma. *Onco Targets Ther.* **2016**, *9*, 2297–2304. [CrossRef] [PubMed]

35. Kim, D.J.; Lee, J.H.; Park, H.R.; Choi, Y.W. Acetylshikonin inhibits growth of oral squamous cell carcinoma by inducing apoptosis. *Arch. Oral Biol.* **2016**, *70*, 149–157. [CrossRef] [PubMed]

36. Liu, C.M.; Peng, C.Y.; Liao, Y.W.; Lu, M.Y.; Tsai, M.L.; Yeh, J.C.; Yu, C.H.; Yu, C.C. Sulforaphane targets cancer stemness and tumor initiating properties in oral squamous cell carcinomas via mir-200c induction. *J. Formos. Med. Assoc.* **2017**, *116*, 41–48. [CrossRef] [PubMed]

37. Su, N.W.; Wu, S.H.; Chi, C.W.; Liu, C.J.; Tsai, T.H.; Chen, Y.J. Metronomic cordycepin therapy prolongs survival of oral cancer-bearing mice and inhibits epithelial-mesenchymal transition. *Molecules* **2017**, *22*, 629. [CrossRef] [PubMed]

38. Kwak, H.H.; Kim, I.R.; Kim, H.J.; Park, B.S.; Yu, S.B. Alpha-mangostin induces apoptosis and cell cycle arrest in oral squamous cell carcinoma cell. *Evid. Based Complement. Altern. Med.* **2016**, *2016*, e5352412. [CrossRef] [PubMed]

39. Tjioe, K.C.; Tostes Oliveira, D.; Gavard, J. Luteolin impacts on the DNA damage pathway in oral squamous cell carcinoma. *Nutr. Cancer* **2016**, *68*, 838–847. [CrossRef] [PubMed]

40. Utaipan, T.; Athipornchai, A.; Suksamrarn, A.; Jirachotikoon, C.; Yuan, X.; Lertcanawanichakul, M.; Chunglok, W. Carbazole alkaloids from murraya koenigii trigger apoptosis and autophagic flux inhibition in human oral squamous cell carcinoma cells. *J. Nat. Med.* **2017**, *71*, 158–169. [CrossRef] [PubMed]

41. Espona-Fiedler, M.; Soto-Cerrato, V.; Hosseini, A.; Lizcano, J.M.; Guallar, V.; Quesada, R.; Gao, T.; Perez-Tomas, R. Identification of dual mtorc1 and mtorc2 inhibitors in melanoma cells: Prodigiosin vs. Obatoclax. *Biochem. Pharmacol.* **2012**, *83*, 489–496. [CrossRef] [PubMed]

42. Smithen, D.A.; Forrester, A.M.; Corkery, D.P.; Dellaire, G.; Colpitts, J.; McFarland, S.A.; Berman, J.N.; Thompson, A. Investigations regarding the utility of prodigiosenes to treat leukemia. *Org. Biomol. Chem.* **2013**, *11*, 62–68. [CrossRef] [PubMed]

43. Alexandrova, E.M.; Yallowitz, A.R.; Li, D.; Xu, S.; Schulz, R.; Proia, D.A.; Lozano, G.; Dobbelstein, M.; Moll, U.M. Improving survival by exploiting tumour dependence on stabilized mutant p53 for treatment. *Nature* **2015**, *523*, 352–356. [CrossRef] [PubMed]

44. Kim, J.; Kundu, M.; Viollet, B.; Guan, K.L. Ampk and mtor regulate autophagy through direct phosphorylation of ulk1. *Nat. Cell Biol.* **2011**, *13*, 132–141. [CrossRef] [PubMed]

45. Mihaylova, M.M.; Shaw, R.J. The ampk signalling pathway coordinates cell growth, autophagy and metabolism. *Nat. Cell Biol.* **2011**, *13*, 1016–1023. [CrossRef] [PubMed]

46. Funderburk, S.F.; Wang, Q.J.; Yue, Z. The beclin 1-vps34 complex—At the crossroads of autophagy and beyond. *Trends Cell Biol.* **2010**, *20*, 355–362. [CrossRef] [PubMed]

47. Lee, E.; Lee, C.G.; Yim, J.H.; Lee, H.K.; Pyo, S. Ramalin-mediated apoptosis is enhanced by autophagy inhibition in human breast cancer cells. *Phytother. Res.* **2016**, *30*, 426–438. [CrossRef] [PubMed]

48. Vegliante, R.; Desideri, E.; Di Leo, L.; Ciriolo, M.R. Dehydroepiandrosterone triggers autophagic cell death in human hepatoma cell line hepg2 via jnk-mediated p62/sqstm1 expression. *Carcinogenesis* **2016**, *37*, 233–244. [CrossRef] [PubMed]

49. Jiang, L.C.; Xin, Z.Y.; Deborah, B.; Zhang, J.S.; Yuan, D.Y.; Xu, K.; Liu, X.B.; Jiang, H.Q.; Fan, Q.C.; Zhang, B.; et al. Inhibition of autophagy augments apoptosis in human oral squamous cell carcinoma under nutrient depletion. *J. Oral Pathol. Med.* **2015**, *44*, 361–366. [CrossRef] [PubMed]

50. Xavier, C.P.; Lima, C.F.; Pedro, D.F.; Wilson, J.M.; Kristiansen, K.; Pereira-Wilson, C. Ursolic acid induces cell death and modulates autophagy through jnk pathway in apoptosis-resistant colorectal cancer cells. *J. Nutr. Biochem.* **2013**, *24*, 706–712. [CrossRef] [PubMed]

51. Puissant, A.; Auberger, P. Ampk- and p62/sqstm1-dependent autophagy mediate resveratrol-induced cell death in chronic myelogenous leukemia. *Autophagy* **2010**, *6*, 655–657. [CrossRef] [PubMed]

52. Puissant, A.; Robert, G.; Fenouille, N.; Luciano, F.; Cassuto, J.P.; Raynaud, S.; Auberger, P. Resveratrol promotes autophagic cell death in chronic myelogenous leukemia cells via jnk-mediated p62/sqstm1 expression and ampk activation. *Cancer Res.* **2010**, *70*, 1042–1052. [CrossRef] [PubMed]

53. Utaipan, T.; Athipornchai, A.; Suksamrarn, A.; Chunsrivirot, S.; Chunglok, W. Isomahanine induces endoplasmic reticulum stress and simultaneously triggers p38 mapk-mediated apoptosis and autophagy in multidrug-resistant human oral squamous cell carcinoma cells. *Oncol. Rep.* **2017**, *37*, 1243–1252. [PubMed]

54. Shrotriya, S.; Tyagi, A.; Deep, G.; Orlicky, D.J.; Wisell, J.; Wang, X.J.; Sclafani, R.A.; Agarwal, R.; Agarwal, C. Grape seed extract and resveratrol prevent 4-nitroquinoline 1-oxide induced oral tumorigenesis in mice by modulating ampk activation and associated biological responses. *Mol. Carcinog.* **2015**, *54*, 291–300. [CrossRef] [PubMed]

55. Lee, J.G.; Shin, J.H.; Shim, H.S.; Lee, C.Y.; Kim, D.J.; Kim, Y.S.; Chung, K.Y. Autophagy contributes to the chemoresistance of non-small cell lung cancer in hypoxic conditions. *Respir. Res.* **2015**, *16*, e138. [CrossRef] [PubMed]

56. Ikeda, T.; Ishii, K.A.; Saito, Y.; Miura, M.; Otagiri, A.; Kawakami, Y.; Shimano, H.; Hara, H.; Takekoshi, K. Inhibition of autophagy enhances sunitinib-induced cytotoxicity in rat pheochromocytoma pc12 cells. *J. Pharmacol. Sci.* **2013**, *121*, 67–73. [CrossRef] [PubMed]

57. Huang, S. Inhibition of pi3k/akt/mtor signaling by natural products. *Anticancer Agents Med. Chem.* **2013**, *13*, 967–970. [CrossRef] [PubMed]

58. Park, D.; Jeong, H.; Lee, M.N.; Koh, A.; Kwon, O.; Yang, Y.R.; Noh, J.; Suh, P.-G.; Park, H.; Ryu, S.H. Resveratrol induces autophagy by directly inhibiting mtor through atp competition. *Sci. Rep.* **2016**, *6*, e21772. [CrossRef] [PubMed]

59. Din, F.V.N.; Valanciute, A.; Houde, V.P.; Zibrova, D.; Green, K.A.; Sakamoto, K.; Alessi, D.R.; Dunlop, M.G. Aspirin inhibits mtor signaling, activates amp-activated protein kinase, and induces autophagy in colorectal cancer cells. *Gastroenterology* **2012**, *142*, 1504–1515. [CrossRef] [PubMed]

60. Wu, Y.-T.; Tan, H.-L.; Shui, G.; Bauvy, C.; Huang, Q.; Wenk, M.R.; Ong, C.-N.; Codogno, P.; Shen, H.-M. Dual role of 3-methyladenine in modulation of autophagy via different temporal patterns of inhibition on class i and iii phosphoinositide 3-kinase. *J. Biol. Chem.* **2010**, *285*, 10850–10861. [CrossRef] [PubMed]

61. White, E.; Karp, C.; Strohecker, A.M.; Guo, Y.; Mathew, R. Role of autophagy in suppression of inflammation and cancer. *Curr. Opin. Cell Biol.* **2010**, *22*, 212–217. [CrossRef] [PubMed]

62. Hassankhani, R.; Sam, M.R.; Esmaeilou, M.; Ahangar, P. Prodigiosin isolated from cell wall of *serratia marcescens* alters expression of apoptosis-related genes and increases apoptosis in colorectal cancer cells. *Med. Oncol.* **2015**, *32*, 366–374. [CrossRef] [PubMed]

63. Cosway, B.; Lovat, P. The role of autophagy in squamous cell carcinoma of the head and neck. *Oral Oncol.* **2016**, *54*, 1–6. [CrossRef] [PubMed]

64. Liu, J.L.; Chen, F.F.; Lung, J.; Lo, C.H.; Lee, F.H.; Lu, Y.C.; Hung, C.H. Prognostic significance of p62/sqstm1 subcellular localization and lc3b in oral squamous cell carcinoma. *Br. J. Cancer* **2014**, *111*, 944–954. [CrossRef] [PubMed]

65. Zhang, J.; Shen, Y.; Liu, J.; Wei, D. Antimetastatic effect of prodigiosin through inhibition of tumor invasion. *Biochem. Pharmacol.* **2005**, *69*, 407–414. [CrossRef] [PubMed]

66. Prabhu, V.V.; Hong, B.; Allen, J.E.; Zhang, S.; Lulla, A.R.; Dicker, D.T.; El-Deiry, W.S. Small-molecule prodigiosin restores p53 tumor suppressor activity in chemoresistant colorectal cancer stem cells via c-jun-mediated δnp73 inhibition and p73 activation. *Cancer Res.* **2016**, *76*, 1989–1999. [CrossRef] [PubMed]

67. Wang, Z.; Li, B.; Zhou, L.; Yu, S.; Su, Z.; Song, J.; Sun, Q.; Sha, O.; Wang, X.; Jiang, W.; et al. Prodigiosin inhibits wnt/β-catenin signaling and exerts anticancer activity in breast cancer cells. *Proc. Natl. Acad. Sci. USA* **2016**, *113*, 13150–13155. [CrossRef] [PubMed]

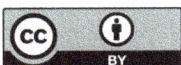

Article

Pharmacokinetics of Jaspine B and Enhancement of Intestinal Absorption of Jaspine B in the Presence of Bile Acid in Rats

Min-Koo Choi [1], Jihoon Lee [2], So Jeong Nam [2], Yun Ju Kang [2], Youjin Han [2], Kwangik Choi [2], Young A. Choi [1], Mihwa Kwon [2], Dongjoo Lee [3] and Im-Sook Song [2,*]

[1] College of Pharmacy, Dankook University, Cheon-an 31116, Korea; minkoochoi@dankook.ac.kr (M.-K.C.); ayha06@gmail.com (Y.A.C.)
[2] College of Pharmacy and Research Institute of Pharmaceutical Sciences, Kyungpook National University, Daegu 41566, Korea; legadema0905@naver.com (J.L.); goddns159@nate.com (S.J.N.); yun-ju6895@nate.com (Y.J.K.); gksdbwls2@nate.com (Y.H.); reggirchoi@naver.com (K.C.); mihwa_k@naver.com (M.K.)
[3] College of Pharmacy, Ajou University, Suwon 16499, Korea; dongjoo@ajou.ac.kr
* Correspondence: isssong@knu.ac.kr; Tel.: +82-53-950-8575; Fax: +82-53-950-8557

Received: 13 July 2017; Accepted: 30 August 2017; Published: 1 September 2017

Abstract: We aimed to investigate the pharmacokinetics and the underlying mechanisms of the intestinal absorption, distribution, metabolism, and excretion of Jaspine B in rats. The oral bioavailability of Jaspine B was 6.2%, but it decreased to 1.6% in bile-depleted rats and increased to 41.2% (normal) and 23.5% (bile-depleted) with taurocholate supplementation (60 mg/kg). Consistent with the increased absorption in the presence of bile salts, rat intestinal permeability of Jaspine B also increased in the presence of 10 mM taurocholate or 20% bile. Further studies demonstrated that the enhanced intestinal permeability with bile salts was due to increased lipophilicity and decreased membrane integrity. Jaspine B was designated as a highly tissue-distributed compound, because it showed large tissue to plasma ratios in the brain, kidney, heart, and spleen. Moreover, the recovery of Jaspine B from the feces and urine after an intravenous administration was about 6.3%, suggesting a substantial metabolism of Jaspine B. Consistent with this observation, 80% of the administered Jaspine B was degraded after 1 h incubation with rat liver microsomes. In conclusion, the facilitated intestinal permeability in the presence of bile salts could significantly increase the bioavailability of Jaspine B and could lead to the development of oral formulations of Jaspine B with bile salts. Moreover, the highly distributed features of Jaspine B in the brain, kidney, heart, and spleen should be carefully considered in the therapeutic effect and toxicity of this compound.

Keywords: Jaspine B; bile salts; intestinal permeability; bioavailability; metabolic instability

1. Introduction

The development of anticancer drugs with effective therapeutic mechanisms is most interesting [1]. In that sense, various herbal and marine compounds have emerged as potential alternative medicines because of their structural diversity and safety, which was demonstrated by their long history of dietary use [2,3]. Marine natural products have been isolated since 1950s and marine sponges are one of the richest sources of bioactive compounds, showing the anti-proliferative effect through the inhibition of microtubule formation, the promotion of cell growth arrest, and stimulation of the cells death program [1]. Of these, the discovery of the sponge-derived nucleoside such as spongothymidine and spongouridine was made and three marine-based, anti-cancer drugs are currently being marketed [4]. Cytarabine was the first marine-derived anticancer drug approved in 1998 for the treatment of acute myelogenous leukemia. It was isolated from the marine sponge, Cryptotethya crypta, and induced apoptotic signals by inhibiting the NF-κB/Rel nuclear factor and binding to Bcl-2, and resulting in growth arrest at the G1/S phase [5]. Trabectedin, isolated from Ecteinascidia turbinata, was an approved anti-cancer drug against metastatic soft tissue carcinoma and ovarian cancer in 2009 in Europe [1]. Another approved marine drug is eribulin, an analog of halichondrin B, extracted from the marine sponge, Halichondria okadai [6], in 2010 from the FDA for the treatment of metastatic breast cancer. It also showed Bcl-2 inactivation and inhibition of microtubule polymerization [1,6].

Metabolites of sphingolipids such as ceramide, sphingosine, and sphingosine-1-phosphate (S1P), have been emerged as modulators for cancer progression [7]. Several studies addressing the effectiveness of sphingosine kinase SphK1 inhibition for cancer therapy have been reported [8–11]. The mRNA levels of SphK1 were significantly increased in breast, colon, lung, ovary, uterus, and kidney cancer patients, as well as in acute leukemia patients [12–14], and the downregulation of SphK1 decreased the epidermal growth factor and reduced prolactin- and E2-induced migration in metastatic breast cancer [7].

Jaspine B (pachastrissamine) (Figure 1) is an anhydrophytosphingosine, which is extracted from the marine sponge, *Pachastrissa* spp. [15]. It showed effective anti-cancer activity against several human carcinomas. Owing to its structural similarity with sphingosine, Jaspine B inactivated SphK1 and induced apoptotic signals [16]. In addition, Jaspine B inhibited melanoma cell growth by inhibiting the phosphorylation of Forkhead box O3 (FOXO3) [17] and by inducing apoptosis [18].

Previously, we had reported the anti-tumor activity of Jaspine B against various tumor cells that overexpressed sphingosine kinase. The results showed that Jaspine B was the most effective against breast cancer cells (MCF-7, IC_{50} = 2.31 μM) and showed differential cytotoxicity towards human breast adenocarcinoma (MDA-MB-231, IC_{50} > 100 μM), renal carcinoma (786-O, IC_{50} = 29.4 μM), melanoma (MDA-MB-435, IC_{50} = 2.60 μM), ovarian (SK-OV3, IC_{50} = 4.78 μM), and hepatoma (HepG2, IC_{50} = 5.69 μM) cells. The steady-state cellular concentration of Jaspine B was associated with the cytotoxic effect [19].

However, there have been few studies determining the absorption, disposition, and pharmacokinetic properties of Jaspine B, despite the importance of understanding these properties of the active, natural components. Therefore, in this study, we aimed to evaluate the pharmacokinetics, absorption, disposition, and excretion profile of Jaspine B and to investigate the underlying mechanisms related to its pharmacokinetic properties.

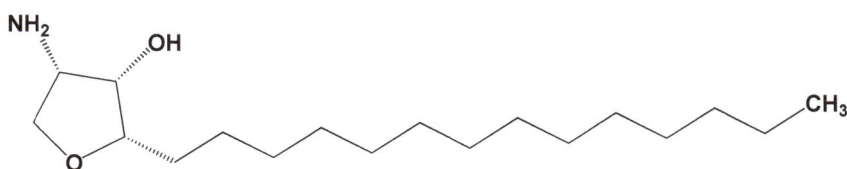

Figure 1. Structure of Jaspine B.

2. Results

2.1. LC/MS-MS Analysis of Jaspine B in the Biological Samples

We developed an analytical method of Jaspine B in the rat plasma, urine, bile, and various tissue homogenates using a liquid chromatography tandem-mass spectrometry (LC-MS/MS) system. Figure 2A showed the representative multiple reaction monitoring (MRM) chromatograms obtained from the analysis of blank rat plasma and rat plasma samples at 1 h after the oral dose of 30 mg/kg Jaspine B. In addition, representative MRM chromatograms obtained from other resources such as urine, bile, and tissue homogenates of brain, kidney, liver, heart, and spleen were also shown in Figure 2B–H. Although the concentration range of Jaspine B varied depending on the biological samples used, the analyses of Jaspine B in other resources such as urine, bile, and tissue homogenates of brain, kidney, liver, heart, and spleen did not show any interference at the retention times of Jaspine B (Figure 2).

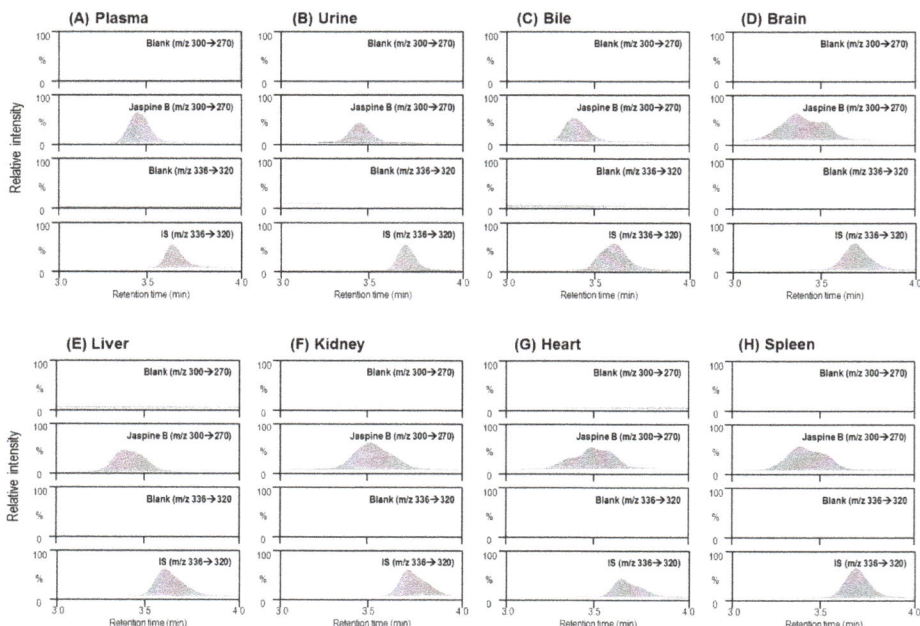

Figure 2. Representative multiple reaction monitoring (MRM) chromatograms of rat (**A**) plasma, (**B**) urine, (**C**) bile, and tissue homogenates of (**D**) brain, (**E**) liver, (**F**) kidney, (**G**) heart, and (**H**) spleen samples. In each panel from A to H, the chromatograms represent the MRM of Jaspine B (m/z 300→270) and internal standard (IS) (berberine, m/z 336→320) from blank and biological samples, respectively.

2.2. Pharmacokinetics of Jaspine B Following Intravenous Injection of 10 mg/kg Jaspine B

The mean plasma concentration–time profiles of Jaspine B after IV administration at a dose of 10 mg/kg in rats are shown in Figure 3A and the relevant pharmacokinetic parameters are listed in Table 1. The plasma concentration of Jaspine B after a IV administration declined, with a bi-exponential elimination process, and the terminal half-life was calculated as 6.7 h. The distribution half-life, which was calculated from the distribution phase in Figure 3A, was 1.4 h, and the volume of distribution at steady-state was calculated as 21.2 L/kg, suggesting a fast distribution of this compound into the second compartment.

The excreted amounts of Jaspine B via the urinary and biliary routes are shown in Figure 3B. After 10 mg/kg of Jaspine B was administered, $0.4 \pm 0.2\%$ and $2.4 \pm 0.8\%$ of the IV dose were recovered in the urine and bile, respectively (Table 1), suggesting that there was substantial metabolism of Jaspine B during its disposition. This was also supported by the large systemic clearance (CL_{total}) of Jaspine B, 98.3 mL/min/kg and low CL_{bile} and CL_{urine} of Jaspine B compared with CL_{total}. The contribution of CL_{bile} and CL_{urine} was about 4% of CL_{total} (Table 1).

Table 1. Pharmacokinetic parameters of Jaspine B after intravenous injection of Jaspine B at a dose of 10 mg/kg in rats.

	Parameters	IV (10 mg/kg)
Plasma	$T_{1/2}$ (h)	6.7 ± 1.6
	MRT (h)	3.6 ± 0.5
	AUC_{12h} (ng·h/mL)	1286.9 ± 165.6
	AUC_{∞} (ng·h/mL)	1701.9 ± 137.1
	Vss (L/kg)	21.2 ± 2.6
	CL_{total} (mL/min/kg)	98.3 ± 7.7
Bile	X_{bile} (% of dose)	2.4 ± 0.8
	CL_{bile} (mL/min/kg)	3.1 ± 0.6
Urine	X_{urine} (% of dose)	0.4 ± 0.2
	CL_{urine} (mL/min/kg)	0.5 ± 0.3

Data are expressed as the means ± S.D. from four different rats.

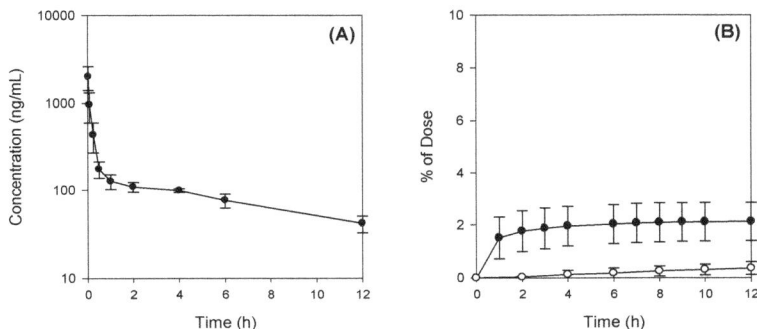

Figure 3. (**A**) Plasma concentration-time profile and (**B**) biliary (●) and urinary (○) excretion of Jaspine B after intravenous injection of Jaspine B (10 mg/kg) in rats. The means ± S.D. from four different rats.

The cumulative excreted amounts of Jaspine B were measured for 72 h using a metabolic cage. After 10 mg/kg of Jaspine B was intravenously administered, 1.6 ± 0.7% and 4.7 ± 0.8% of the dose were recovered after 72 h from the urine and feces, respectively. Therefore, over the 72 h period, the recovery of unaltered Jaspine B was estimated to be 6.3% of the single IV dose from the combined feces and urine samples, suggesting that a large amount of Jaspine B was metabolized in vivo.

2.3. Metabolic Instability of Jaspine B

Given the evidence of the substantial metabolism of Jaspine B, its microsomal stability was measured using rat liver microsomes. The percentage remaining after incubating for 30 min and 60 min was 59.8% and 20.4%, respectively, and the degradation half-life was calculated as 24 min (Figure 4). These results suggest the metabolic instability of Jaspine B in the liver, which is consistent with the previous results of the low contribution of biliary and urinary excretion of Jaspine B to the large clearance of this compound.

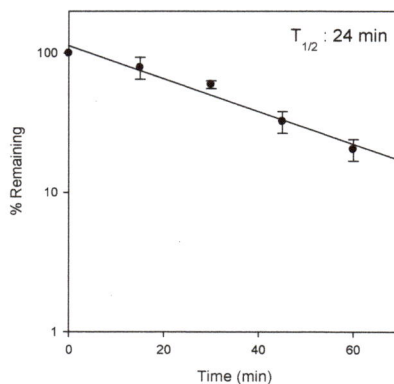

Figure 4. Metabolic instability of Jaspine B with rat liver microsomes. Jaspine B (1 μM) was incubated with 0.25 mg rat liver microsomes in the presence of a β-nicotinamide adenine dinucleotide 2′-phosphate reduced (NADPH)-generating system (1.3 mM β-NADP, 3.3 mM glucose-6-phosphate, 3.3 mM MgCl$_2$, and 1.0 unit/mL glucose-6-phosphate dehydrogenase) for 60 min at 37 °C in a shaking water bath. The half-life (T$_{1/2}$) was calculated from the first-order degradation rate constant.

2.4. Bile Acid Facilitates the Intestinal Absorption of Jaspine B

The mean plasma concentration–time profiles of Jaspine B after oral administration at a dose of 30 mg/kg in rats are shown in Figure 5A, and the relevant pharmacokinetic parameters are listed in control group (Table 2). Absolute bioavailability (BA), calculated by dividing the oral AUC by the intravenous AUC, was calculated as 6.2%.

Interestingly, the plasma concentration of Jaspine B decreased in the rats with bile depletion (Figure 5B) compared with that of the control group (Figure 5A). In our study, bile depletion was accomplished with 4 h drainage of bile through the bile cannula, which was cannulated to the bile duct using PE-10 tubing. After this bile drainage, the concentration of total bile salts in the bile sample decreased from 50.1 ± 6.5 mM to 15.3 ± 5.7 mM (i.e., 70% decrease), which was measured using an enzymatic-fluorometric assay with the slight modifications reported by Choi et al. [20].

However, the co-administration of taurocholate (TC, 60 mg/kg) with Jaspine B in bile-depleted rats prevented the decrease in plasma Jaspine B and elevated the levels above those of controls (Figure 5C). This was also observed when TC was administered to the control rats; in this situation, the plasma concentration of Jaspine B was higher than that of the control group (Figure 5D vs. Figure 5A). The addition of TC increased the C$_{max}$ and AUC of orally administered Jaspine B without changing the terminal half-life (T$_{1/2}$) (Table 2). These results suggest that the increase in C$_{max}$ and AUC by the addition of TC was attributed to the absorption phase rather than the disposition phase, and consequently, the addition of TC increased the oral bioavailability of this compound from 6.2% to 41.2% (Table 2). In case of bile-depleted rats, AUC$_\infty$ and T$_{1/2}$ were not calculated because the elimination rate constant could not be obtained. Therefore, the oral bioavailability of Jaspine B was calculated as AUC$_{12h,PO}$/AUC$_{12h,IV}$.

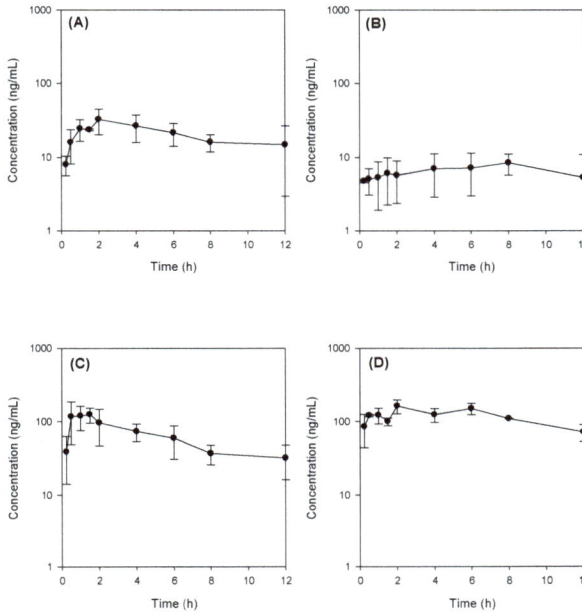

Figure 5. Plasma concentration-time profile of Jaspine B in rats after oral administration of Jaspine B (30 mg/kg) with or without taurocholate (TC; 60 mg/kg) in control and bile-depleted rats. (**A**) Control group; (**B**) bile-depleted group; (**C**) bile-depletion + TC; (**D**) Control + TC group. Data are expressed as the means ± S.D. from three to five different rats.

Table 2. Pharmacokinetic parameters of Jaspine B after oral administration of Jaspine B at a dose of 30 mg/kg in rats.

Parameters	Control (*n* = 3)	Bile Depletion (*n* = 3)	Bile Depletion + TC (*n* = 5)	Control + TC (*n* = 3)
C_{max} (ng/mL)	36.3 ± 11.3	8.5 ± 2.8 *	163.4 ± 28.4 *	174.1 ± 13.0 *
T_{max} (h)	2.5 ± 1.3	9.3 ± 2.3 *	1.0 ± 0.5	3.3 ± 2.3
$T_{1/2}$ (h)	5.5 ± 1.1	–	7.2 ± 1.5	6.4 ± 2.8
MRT (h)	4.9 ± 0.4	6.1 ± 0.3 *	4.9 ± 0.5	5.5 ± 0.03
AUC_{12h} (ng·h/mL)	240.6 ± 57.8	80.3 ± 42.7 *	828.3 ± 180 *	1406.3 ± 4.3 *,#
AUC_∞ (ng·h/mL)	314.4 ± 76.1	–	1201.7 ± 254 *	2100.9 ± 419 *,#
BA (%)	6.2	1.6	23.5	41.2

Each value represents the mean ± S.D. * $p < 0.05$, significant versus control group; # $p < 0.05$, significant versus Bile depletion + TC group.

To confirm the role of bile salts in intestinal absorption, we measured intestinal permeability in rat intestinal segments using an Ussing chamber system. At first, to determine the optimized bile salt concentration, we monitored the permeability of Lucifer yellow, a marker compound for paracellular permeation and cell integrity [21,22], with various concentrations of TC (0.1–100 mM). The permeability of Lucifer yellow increased gradually until 10 mM TC and then showed a sharp increase at 100 mM TC (Figure 6A), suggesting that the cell integrity was disrupted between 10 and 100 mM TC.

To determine whether the intestinal absorption was increased by the addition of 10 mM TC, we measured the absorptive (A to B direction) and secretory (B to A direction) permeability of Jaspine B with 10 mM TC. The addition of 10 mM TC increased both absorptive and secretory permeability approximately 5-fold. The increased Jaspine B permeability (~5-fold) was greater than the increased Lucifer yellow permeability caused by tight junction opening (~2.8-fold), which was 56% of the increased Jaspine B permeability (Figure 6B). Therefore, the facilitated intestinal permeability in the presence of TC was caused partly by tight junction opening and partly by another unidentified mechanism. Since the absorptive and secretory permeabilities were almost identical, the intestinal transport mechanism such as efflux pump or uptake transport process may not contribute to the intestinal absorption of this compound [23]. The addition of 20% bile also increased the permeability of Jaspine B (Figure 6B) where the concentration of total bile salts in 20% bile was 10.1 ± 2.3 mM, which is similar to the concentration of bile salts in the intestinal lumen [24] as well as equivalent to 10 mM TC. Thus the increased Jaspine B permeability in the presence of 10 mM TC and 20% bile was not statistically different.

Next, to unveil other mechanisms of increased Jaspine B permeability, we investigated whether the lipophilicity of Jaspine B increased in the presence of TC, since tertiary amines and quaternary ammonium can interact with endogenous bile to form lipophilic ion-pair complexes of Jaspine B and TC [25–27]. The partition coefficient of Jaspine B increased 10-fold in the presence of 10 mM TC compared with that in the absence of TC (Figure 6C).

Collectively, these results show that the enhancement of Jaspine B absorption in the presence of 20% bile and 10 mM TC could be attributed to the increased passive diffusion by the formation of lipophilic ion-pair complexes of Jaspine B-bile salts, as well as increased paracellular permeation through the tight junction opening by bile or bile salts [22,25]. As consequence, the increased absorption of Jaspine B in the presence of bile salts would lead to the increased BA of Jaspine B.

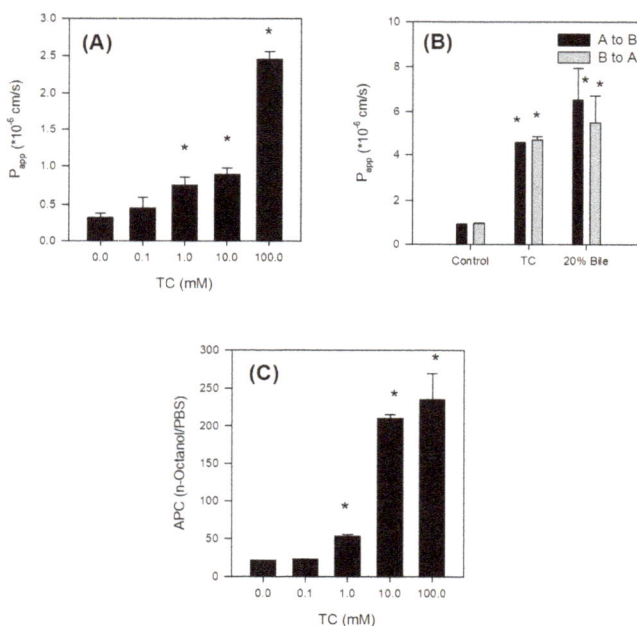

Figure 6. (**A**) Effect of taurocholate (TC) on the permeability of Lucifer yellow in the rat ileum. Permeability (P_{app}) of Lucifer yellow (10 μM) in the presence of TC (0, 0.1, 1, 10, and 100 mM) was measured in the rat ileum using the Ussing chamber system. (**B**) Effect of TC and bile on the permeability of Jaspine B in the rat ileum. Permeability (P_{app}) of Jaspine B (10 μM) in the presence of TC (10 mM) and bile (20%) was measured in the rat ileum using the Ussing chamber system. (**C**) Effect of TC on the lipophilicity of Jaspine B. Apparent partition coefficient (APC) of Jaspine B between *n*-octanol and PBS phases was measured in the presence of TC (0, 0.1, 1, 10, or 100 mM). Each data point represents the mean ± S.D. of three independent experiments. * $p < 0.05$, statistically significant versus the corresponding control group.

2.5. Tissue Distribution of Jaspine B

To investigate the tissue distribution of Jaspine B, its concentrations in the brain, liver, kidney, heart, spleen, and plasma were measured at 0.5 h and 12 h after IV administration of 10 mg/kg. The liver, kidney, heart, and spleen were selected as major organs that show high distribution, and the brain was selected as an organ that shows limited distribution. To calculate the drug concentration ratios of tissue to plasma (T/P ratio) of Jaspine B, 0.5 h and 12 h were selected to represent the distribution and elimination phases, respectively. As shown in Figure 7, the T/P ratios of Jaspine B in the brain, kidney, heart, and spleen were significantly higher than that in the plasma at 0.5 h (i.e., 6.2-, 11.1-, 14.4-, and 18.5-fold greater in the brain, kidney, heart, and spleen, respectively, than in the plasma). The significantly higher concentrations of Jaspine B in the brain, kidney, heart, and spleen were maintained 12 h after administration (i.e., 1.8-, 4.7-, 3.2-, and 3.9-fold greater in the brain, kidney, heart, and spleen, respectively, than in the plasma). These results were consistent with the large volume of distribution of Jaspine B, 21.2 L/kg. Interestingly, the concentration of Jaspine B in the liver was lower than in the other tissues (i.e., 2.3- and 1.2-fold higher than plasma levels at 0.5 and 12 h, respectively), which may be attributed to the substantial metabolism of this compound in the liver.

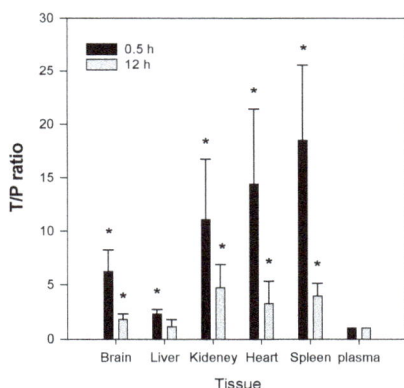

Figure 7. Tissue to plasma (T/P) ratios of Jaspine B recovered from tissues at 0.5 h and 12 h after intravenous (10 mg/kg) administration of Jaspine B to rats. At 0.5 h and 12 h after dosing, plasma, liver, kidney, heart, spleen, and brain samples were collected and the concentrations of Jaspine B in the samples were measured. The bars represent the means ± S.D. of the results from four rats. * $p < 0.05$, significant versus plasma ratio.

3. Discussion

Jaspine B is an anhydrophytosphingosine, extracted from the marine sponge, *Pachastrissa* spp. It shows meaningful inhibitory activity against sphingosine kinases (SphK1 and SphK2), which is an important mechanism of action for its anti-proliferative effect [28]. Jaspine B shows differential efficacy against a variety of tumor types of different tissue origins, and the cellular accumulation of Jaspine B at steady-state is a crucial determining factor of efficacy [19]. Moreover, the intravenous injection of Jaspine B (200 mg/mouse, equivalent to 6.7 mg/kg) on 4th, 8th, and 12th day dramatically decreased metastatic melanoma cell growth in the lungs of Jaspine B-injected mice on day 14 [18]. Although this in vivo and in vitro anti-proliferative effects of Jaspine B, the pharmacokinetics features of this compound was not investigated.

Therefore, the next step in understanding the anti-tumor activity of Jaspine B was to investigate its pharmacokinetic characteristics and the underlying mechanisms controlling the absorption, distribution, metabolism, and elimination of this compound.

The absorption of Jaspine B itself was limited, however, and the presence of bile salts increased the intestinal permeability of this compound over 5-fold by increasing partitioning of Jaspine B to lipophilic phase and tight junction opening (Figure 6). However, since the TC infusion to the rat liver did not significantly alter the metabolic activity of sulfobromophthalein [29], it is unlikely to conclude that concomitant administration of Jaspine B with TC inhibited metabolism of Jaspine B, and consequently increased BA of Jaspine B. To the contrary, the co-existence of Jaspine B with TC increased intestinal permeability and thereby increased the intestinal absorption and BA of Jaspine B. The results were consistent with a low oral BA of Jaspine B (6.2%) that decreased to 1.6% in bile-depleted rats, and after the co-addition of TC, oral BA increased to 23.5% in bile-depleted rats and 41.2% in control rats. Since the increased permeability of Jaspine B was the modulating factor that increased the low oral BA of Jaspine B and the permeability of Jaspine B in the rat intestine was very limited (0.11×10^{-6} cm/s), the important factors for the low BA of Jaspine B can be elucidated as low intestinal permeability. In addition, the low oral BA was known to be attributed to the limited permeability, the chemical and enzymatic degradation of a drug in the gut lumen, and the intestinal or hepatic first-pass effect [30]. The instability of Jaspine B in the gut lumen and the hepatic or intestinal first-pass effect also need to be investigated to elucidate the underlying mechanisms for the low BA of Jaspine B.

In our study, bile depletion was accomplished with 4 h drainage of bile through the bile cannula, which was evidenced by the 70% reduction of total bile salts concentration (from 50.1 ± 6.5 mM in control rats to 15.3 ± 5.7 mM) in bile drainage rats, which we named as bile-depleted rats. Since over 90% of bile salts were recirculated gut-liver-bile cycle [31], a 70% decrease of bile salts concentration in the bile implicated the significant decrease of bile salts in the gut as well, which resulted in the decreased absorption of Jaspine B in bile-depleted rats (Figure 5B). As a result of TC supplementation (60 mg/kg) with Jaspine B, which was suspended in 3 mL of DMSO: PEG400: saline solution, the TC concentration would be approximately 10 mM in the gut and could enhance the absorption of Jaspine B in rats from bile depletion + TC group and control + TC group (Figure 5C,D).

These results could be applied to the development of oral Jaspine B formulations consisting of bile salts and lipophilic phospholipids, i.e., mixed micelle formulations [32], to increase the permeability and lipophilicity of this compound. However, for the clinical and pharmaceutical application, the use of pharmaceutical excipients that enhance the transport without affecting tight junctions of intestine rather than high concentrations of TC would be the best approach. For example, SP1049C (Supratek Pharma Inc., Montreal, PQ, Canada), a doxorubicin-containing mixed-micelle formulation with Pluronic L61 and F127, showed increased cellular concentration of the doxorubicin in tumor cells and has reached clinical phase 3 study because of its superior antitumor activity compared with that of doxorubicin standard formulation [33]. A phospholipid-Tween 80 mixed micelle formulation of paclitaxel showed higher anti-tumor activity and reduced systemic toxicity than Taxol formulation did [34].

The second feature of Jaspine B is that it is highly distributed to tissues such as brain, kidney, heart, and spleen. The T/P ratios in these organs were 6.2, 11.1, 14.4, and 18.5, respectively, and remained elevated 2–4-fold 12 h after a single IV administration of Jaspine B (Figure 7). Since we previously reported that the steady-state drug concentration was important for the anti-cancer efficacy of this compound [19,35,36], the tissue distribution of Jaspine B is very important to predict the therapeutic efficacy of this compound. Moreover, this compound showed differential cytotoxicity depending on the cancer cell type, thus the highly tissue distributed features of this compound should be carefully considered in terms of drug response and toxicity. However, we should note that the use of PEG400 as a vehicle in the tissue distribution study (Figure 7) might change the tissue distribution profile of Jaspine B because PEG400 has an ability to entrap of this compound in the spleen's reticuloendothelial systems and thereby increase the in vivo metabolic stability compared with in vitro metabolic stability results (Figure 4).

In addition, the low the recovery from feces and urine (about 6.3% after IV administration) was consistent with the observed microsomal instability in the rat liver microsomes (Figure 4), although the involvement CYP enzymes as well as the proposed metabolite structures were not investigated in this study. Therefore, identification of metabolites and the elucidation of the metabolic enzyme(s) involved will be necessary for future investigation. Moreover, since the metabolites of Jaspine B may have pharmacological activities on the inhibition of SphK1 and the inhibition of FOXO3 phosphorylaiton, the evaluation of the pharmacological activity or toxicity of the proposed metabolite would be of importance.

4. Materials and Methods

4.1. Reagents

Jaspine B was synthesized by Dr. D. Lee (Ajou University, Suwon, Korea) with a purity of over 99% and was confirmed by nuclear magnetic resonance (NMR) and mass spectroscopy results [37]. Its structure is shown in Figure 1.

Hank's balanced salt solution (HBSS), taurocholate (TC), Lucifer yellow, dimethyl sulfoxide (DMSO), polyethylene glycol (PEG) 400, β-nicotinamide adenine dinucleotide (β-NAD), 3α-hydroxysteroid dehydrogenase (3α-HSD), EDTA, and Tris base were purchased from Sigma-Aldrich (St. Louis, MO, USA). Fetal bovine serum, Dulbecco's Modified Eagle's medium (DMEM), and penicillin-streptomycin were purchased from Hyclone Laboratories (Logan, UT, USA). All other reagents were reagent grade.

Rat liver microsomes (RLMs) from Sprague Dawley (SD) rats and the reaction solutions, including the NADH-generating system were purchased from BD-Corning (Corning, NY, USA).

A NaviCyte Ussing chamber system was obtained from Harvard Apparatus Co. (Holliston, MA, USA). Round metabolic cages for rats were purchased from Jungdo B&P Inc. (Seoul, Korea).

4.2. LC-MS/MS Analysis of Jaspine B

The concentrations of Jaspine B in the biological samples were analyzed using an Agilent 6430 Triple Quad LC/MS-MS system (Agilent, Wilmington, DE, USA) coupled with an Agilent Infinity 1290 series high performance liquid chromatography (HPLC) system. The separation was performed on a Synergi Polar RP column (2.0 mm i.d.× 150 mm, 4 μm, Phenomenex) using a mobile phase that consisted of acetonitrile and DDW (85:15, v/v) with 0.1% formic acid at a flow rate of 0.2 mL/min. Mass spectra were recorded by electrospray ionization in the positive mode. Quantification was performed using multiple reaction monitoring (MRM) at m/z 300.3→270.2 for Jaspine B and m/z 336.1→320.0 for berberine.

For the analytical validation of Jaspine B in plasma samples, the standard curve range was 25–5000 ng/mL and the concentrations of quality control (QC) samples were 75, 500, and 3000 ng/mL. The recovery of these spiked QC sample were in the range of 88.2–98.1%. Intra- and inter-day precision and accuracy had coefficients of variance of less than 10%. The stability of Jaspine B QC samples after 3 freeze thaw cycles were 83.9–94.4% and the short-term stability of these samples after standing for 6 h at room temperature was 94.3–100.1%.

The respective standard curve range and sample preparation methods in various biological samples from various experiments were described in detail in each experimental section.

4.3. Pharmacokinetics of Jaspine B

Male SD rats (aged 8–9 weeks, weighing 250–300 g) were obtained from Samtako Bio Korea, Inc. (Osan, Korea). The rats were acclimatized for 1 week in a temperature-controlled room (23 ± 2 °C) with a 12-h illumination cycle. Food and water were given *ad libitum*. All animal procedures were approved by the Animal Care and Use Committee of the Kyungpook National University (No. 2015-0064). The rats were fasted for at least 12 h before the oral administration of drugs.

The femoral artery, femoral vein, and bile duct were cannulated with polyethylene tubes (PE-50 and PE-10; Jungdo, Seoul, Korea) under light anesthesia with isoflurane.

For intravenous (IV) dosing, Jaspine B was dissolved in a vehicle containing DMSO: PEG400: saline (2:4:4, $v/v/v$) and was IV-injected via the femoral vein at 10 mg/kg (vehicle volume, 1 mL/kg). Blood samples were collected from the femoral artery at 0, 0.083, 0.167, 0.25, 0.5, 1, 2, 4, 6, 8, and 12 h following the IV administration of Jaspine B. Bile and urine samples were collected every 2 h for a total of 12 h. After centrifugation of blood samples at 13,200 rpm for 10 min, aliquots of 50 μL of plasma, bile, and urine were stored at −80 °C until the analysis of Jaspine B.

In the experiment using metabolic cages, feces were collected at 12, 24, 48, and 72 h following the IV administration of Jaspine B (10 mg/kg). Aliquots of 50 μL of urine and 10% feces homogenates were stored at −80 °C until the analysis.

Aliquots (50 μL) of plasma, bile, feces homogenates, and urine samples were added to 250 μL of acetonitrile containing 0.5 ng/mL of berberine (an internal standard). After vortexing for 10 min and centrifugation at 13,200 rpm for 5 min, an aliquot (2 μL) of the supernatant was injected directly into the LC-MS/MS system. For the analysis of plasma concentration, the standard curve range was 25–5000 ng/mL and the concentrations of quality control (QC) samples were 75, 500, and 3000 ng/mL, as described previously. Concentrations of Jaspine B in urine, bile, and feces homogenates were 5–300 ng/mL, 20–5000 ng/mL, and 20–5000 ng/mL, respectively. The concentrations of QC samples were 15, 100, and 300 ng/mL for urine samples and 75, 500, and 3000 ng/mL for bile and feces homogenates.

For oral dosing, Jaspine B was dissolved in a vehicle containing DMSO: PEG400: saline (2:4:4, $v/v/v$) and was administered by oral gavages at a single dose of 30 mg/kg of Jaspine B concomitantly with or without 60 mg/kg TC (vehicle volume, 3 mL/kg) to the control and bile-depleted rats. Bile depletion was accomplished with 4 h drainage of bile through the bile cannula, which was cannulated to the bile duct using PE-10 tubing.

Blood samples (approximately 250 μL each) were collected from the femoral artery at 0, 0.25, 0.5, 1, 1.5, 2, 4, 8, and 12 h following the oral administration of Jaspine B. After centrifugation of blood samples at 13,200 rpm for 10 min, plasma samples (50 μL) were collected and stored at −80 °C until the analysis by liquid chromatography tandem-mass spectrometry (LC-MS/MS). Aliquots (50 μL) of plasma samples were added to 250 μL of acetonitrile containing 0.5 ng/mL of berberine (an internal standard). After vortexing for 10 min and centrifugation at 13,200 rpm for 5 min, an aliquot (10 μL) of the supernatant was injected directly into the LC-MS/MS system. The standard curve range was 5–2000 ng/mL and the concentrations of quality control (QC) samples were 60, 300, and 2000 ng/mL. Standard curves showed good linearity ($R^2 > 0.999$) and the interday accuracy and precision was 99.0–105.1% and 0.3–6.9%, respectively.

4.4. Tissue Distribution of Jaspine B

Jaspine B was dissolved in a vehicle containing DMSO: PEG400: saline (2:4:4, $v/v/v$) and IV-injected via the femoral vein at a dose of 10 mg/kg (vehicle volume, 1 mL/kg). Blood samples were collected from the abdominal artery and animals were euthanized at 0.5 h and 12 h after IV dosing. The blood, brain, liver, kidney, heart, and spleen were immediately excised, gently washed with ice-cold saline, and weighed. The tissue samples were homogenized with 9 volumes of saline. Aliquots of 50 μL of tissue homogenates and plasma were stored at −80 °C until the analysis.

Aliquots (50 μL) of plasma and tissue homogenates were added to 250 μL of acetonitrile containing 0.5 ng/mL of berberine. After vortexing for 10 min and centrifugation at 13,200 rpm for 5 min, an aliquot (2 μL) of the supernatant was injected directly into the LC-MS/MS system. For the analysis of plasma and tissue concentration, the standard curves with a range of 5–1000 ng/mL in the blank plasma and 10% bank tissue homogenates from brain, liver, kidney, heart, and spleen were prepared, and the concentrations of quality control (QC) samples of respective plasma and tissue homogenates were 25 and 750 ng/mL. The recovery of these spiked QC samples were in the range of 73.6–112.2% in all tissue homogenates. Intra- and inter-day precision and accuracy had coefficients of variance of less than 15%.

4.5. Metabolic Stability of Jaspine B in Rat Liver Microsomes (RLMs)

Jaspine B (1 μM) was reconstituted in 100 mM potassium phosphate buffer (pH 7.4) containing 0.25 mg of RLMs and was pre-incubated for 5 min at 37 °C. The reaction was initiated by adding an NADPH-generating system (1.3 mM β-NADP, 3.3 mM glucose-6-phosphate, 3.3 mM MgCl$_2$, and 1.0 unit/mL glucose-6-phosphate dehydrogenase) and then incubated (final volume 100 μL) for 0, 15, 30, and 60 min at 37 °C in a shaking water bath. The reaction was stopped by placing the incubation tubes on ice and adding 200 μL of ice-cold acetonitrile containing 0.5 ng/mL of berberine. After vortexing for 10 min and centrifugation at 13,200 rpm for 5 min, 2 μL of the supernatant was injected directly into the LC-MS/MS system. We also determined the metabolic stability of 1 μM propranolol and 1 μM metformin as a positive and negative control, respectively, using the same procedure [38]. The remaining % of propranolol and metformin after 60 min incubation was 12.2% and 63.4% of initial concentration, indicating the feasibility of this system.

4.6. Determination of Bile Salts Concentration in Bile

Total bile salt concentrations in bile samples were determined by means of an enzymatic-fluorometric assay with the slight modification of Choi at al. [20]. Briefly, bile samples were collected. Fifty μL aliquots of standard TC solutions (5, 10, 25, 50, 100, 200 μM), bile samples were added to 950 μL of reaction buffer containing 1mM β-nicotinamide adenine dinucleotide (β-NAD), 50 μU 3α-hydroxysteroid dehyrogenase (3α-HSD), 0.385 mM EDTA and 760 mM Tris (pH 9.5), followed by incubation at 37 °C for 30 min. The reaction was quenched by the addition of 3 mL of ice cold water and the fluorescence was measured at an excitation wavelength of 340 nm and an emission wavelength of 465 nm.

4.7. Determination of the Intestinal Permeability of Jaspine B

For the measurement of the effect of TC on the tight junction of biological membranes, the permeability of 50 μM Lucifer yellow, a marker of paracellular permeation [21], was measured in the presence of TC (0, 0.1, 1, 10, 100 mM). Prior to the experiment, ileal segments from SD rats (about 20 cm) were placed in the chambers and were submerged in fresh, prewarmed (37 °C) HBSS for 15 min for acclimatization. The chambers were continuously bubbled with carbogen gas (5% CO$_2$/ 95% O$_2$) during the experiment. The experiments began by replacing the HBSS with HBSS containing 50 μM Lucifer yellow and various concentrations of TC on the apical side (A) and adding fresh HBSS to the basal side (B). Aliquots (400 μL) of media were withdrawn from the receiver compartment (B) after 0, 20, 40, 60, and 80 min, and the volume of liquid in the receiver compartment was replenished with fresh, prewarmed HBSS after each sampling. Aliquots (200 μL) of all samples were used for the determination of Lucifer yellow concentration. The fluorescence of Lucifer yellow in the samples was measured using a fluorescence spectrophotometer (Infinite 200 PRO, Tecan, Switzerland) with excitation at 425 nm and emission at 535 nm.

A to B and B to A permeability of Jaspine B was measured in the presence of TC and rat bile. One mL of HBSS containing 50 μM Jaspine B and 10 mM TC or 20% bile was added to the donor side and 1 mL of preheated fresh HBSS was added to the receiver side. Aliquots (400 μL) of media were withdrawn at 0, 20, 40, 60, and 80 min from the receiver compartment as described above. Aliquots (50 μL) of all samples were stored at −80 °C until analysis.

Aliquots (50 μL) of all samples were added to 250 μL of acetonitrile containing 0.5 ng/mL of berberine. After vortexing for 10 min and centrifugation at 13,200 rpm for 5 min, 2 μL of the supernatant was injected directly into the LC-MS/MS system.

4.8. Effect of TC on the Lipophilicity of Jaspine B

The effect of TC on the apparent partition coefficients (APC) of Jaspine B between aqueous and organic phases was investigated [26]. *n*-Octanol and phosphate-buffered saline (PBS, pH 7.4) were used as the organic and aqueous phases, respectively, in the partition study. *n*-Octanol and PBS were saturated with respect to one another prior to use. An equal volume of *n*-octanol was added to PBS (5 mL each) containing Jaspine B (10 mM) and TC (0, 0.1, 1, 10, or 100 mM) in a screw-capped test tube, and the mixture was vortexed vigorously for 5 min followed by shaking for 2 h at 25 °C in a temperature-controlled water bath. After standing for 1 h at 25 °C in the water bath, the mixture was separated into two phases by centrifugation at 3000 rpm for 10 min. The concentration of Jaspine B in a 50-μL aliquot of aqueous and organic phase was measured. Briefly, 50 μL of sample was added to 250 μL of acetonitrile containing 0.5 ng/mL of berberine. After vortexing for 10 min and centrifugation at 13,200 rpm for 5 min, an aliquot (2 μL) of the supernatant was injected directly into the LC-MS/MS system. The APC was calculated from the concentration ratio of each compound between the octanol and PBS phases.

4.9. Data Analysis

Pharmacokinetic parameters were determined using a non-compartmental analysis (WinNonlin® 2.0; Pharsight, Mountain View, CA, USA). Maximum plasma concentration (C_{max}) and time to reach C_{max} (T_{max}) values were obtained from plasma concentration-time curves. The area under the plasma concentration–time curve from zero to infinity (AUC) was calculated using the trapezoidal-extrapolation method. For extrapolation, the area from the last data point to infinity was estimated by dividing the terminal-phase rate constant by plasma concentration at the last time point. Oral bioavailability was calculated by dividing AUC_{PO}, which was normalized by Jaspine B dose (30 mg/kg) by AUC_{IV}, which was also normalized by IV dose of Jaspine B (10 mg/kg):

$$BA(\%) = \frac{\frac{AUC_{\infty,PO}}{Dose(30mg/kg)}}{\frac{AUC_{\infty,IV}}{Dose(10mg/kg)}} \times 100 \tag{1}$$

However, in the case of bile-depleted rats, AUC_{∞} and $T_{1/2}$ were not calculated because the elimination rate constant could not be obtained. Therefore, the oral bioavailability of Jaspine B was calculated as follows:

$$BA(\%) = \frac{\frac{AUC_{12h,PO}}{Dose(30mg/kg)}}{\frac{AUC_{12h,IV}}{Dose(10mg/kg)}} \times 100 \tag{2}$$

Total systemic clearance (CL_{total}) was calculated by dividing IV dose by plasma AUC and the apparent volume of distribution at steady-state (Vss) was calculated by multiplying mean residence time (MRT) by CL_{total}. Urinary and biliary clearances of Jaspine B (CL_{urine} and CL_{bile}) were estimated by dividing the total amount of Jaspine B excreted into urine and bile, respectively, for the 0–12 h period by plasma AUC.

The apparent permeability (P_{app}) of the drug was calculated by dividing the initial drug transport rate (dQ/dt, pmol/min) by the initial drug concentration in the donor compartment of the insert (C_o) multiplied by the surface area of the insert (A, cm²) [22]:

$$P_{app} = \frac{dQ}{dt} \times \frac{1}{AC_o} \tag{3}$$

Data are expressed as the means ± standard deviations (S.D.), and statistical significance was determined by *t*-test using SPSS software version 16.1.

Acknowledgments: This work was supported by a grant from the Korea Institute of Planning and Evaluation for Technology in Food, Agriculture, Forestry, and Fisheries (IPET) through Export Promotion Technology Development Program, funded by the Ministry of Agriculture, Food and Rural Affairs (MAFRA) (No 316017-3), Republic of Korea.

Author Contributions: Im-Sook Song and Min-Koo Choi designed the study, performed the experiments, analyzed the data, and wrote the manuscript. Jihoon Lee, So Jeong Nam, Yun Ju Kang, Youjin Han, Kwangik Choi, Young A. Choi, and Mihwa Kwon performed the pharmacokinetics and tissue distribution study and also performed intestinal permeability experiments and analyzed the Jaspine B concentrations from the various samples. Dongjoo Lee synthesized, purified, and confirmed the Jaspine B. All authors reviewed the manuscript.

Conflicts of Interest: The authors have no conflict of interest.

References

1. Indumathy, S.; Dass, C.R. Finding chemo: The search for marine-based pharmaceutical drugs active against cancer. *J. Pharm. Pharmacol.* **2013**, *65*, 1280–1301. [CrossRef] [PubMed]

2. Haefner, B. Drugs from the deep: Marine natural products as drug candidates. *Drug Discov. Today* **2003**, *8*, 536–544. [CrossRef]

3. Sima, P.; Vetvicka, V. Bioactive substances with anti-neoplastic efficacy from marine invertebrates: Porifera and coelenterata. *World J. Clin. Oncol.* **2011**, *2*, 355–361. [CrossRef] [PubMed]

4. Singh, R.; Sharma, M.; Joshi, P.; Rawat, D.S. Clinical status of anti-cancer agents derived from marine sources. *Anticancer Agents Med. Chem.* **2008**, *8*, 603–617. [CrossRef] [PubMed]

5. Russo, P.; Nastrucci, C.; Cesario, A. From the sea to anticancer therapy. *Curr. Med. Chem.* **2011**, *18*, 3551–3562. [CrossRef] [PubMed]

6. Kuznetsov, G.; Towle, M.J.; Cheng, H.; Kawamura, T.; TenDyke, K.; Liu, D.; Kishi, Y.; Yu, M.J.; Littlefield, B.A. Induction of morphological and biochemical apoptosis following prolonged mitotic blockage by halichondrin b macrocyclic ketone analog e7389. *Cancer Res.* **2004**, *64*, 5760–5766. [CrossRef] [PubMed]

7. Shida, D.; Takabe, K.; Kapitonov, D.; Milstien, S.; Spiegel, S. Targeting SphK1 as a new strategy against cancer. *Curr. Drug Targets* **2008**, *9*, 662–673. [CrossRef] [PubMed]

8. Kunkel, G.T.; Maceyka, M.; Milstien, S.; Spiegel, S. Targeting the sphingosine-1-phosphate axis in cancer, inflammation and beyond. *Nat. Rev. Drug Discov.* **2013**, *12*, 688–702. [CrossRef] [PubMed]

9. Lim, K.G.; Gray, A.I.; Pyne, S.; Pyne, N.J. Resveratrol dimers are novel sphingosine kinase 1 inhibitors and affect sphingosine kinase 1 expression and cancer cell growth and survival. *Br. J. Pharmacol.* **2012**, *166*, 1605–1616. [CrossRef] [PubMed]

10. Lim, K.G.; Tonelli, F.; Li, Z.; Lu, X.; Bittman, R.; Pyne, S.; Pyne, N.J. Fty720 analogues as sphingosine kinase 1 inhibitors: Enzyme inhibition kinetics, allosterism, proteasomal degradation, and actin rearrangement in mcf-7 breast cancer cells. *J. Biol. Chem.* **2011**, *286*, 18633–18640. [CrossRef] [PubMed]

11. Pyne, S.; Bittman, R.; Pyne, N.J. Sphingosine kinase inhibitors and cancer: Seeking the golden sword of hercules. *Cancer Res.* **2011**, *71*, 6576–6582. [CrossRef] [PubMed]

12. French, K.J.; Schrecengost, R.S.; Lee, B.D.; Zhuang, Y.; Smith, S.N.; Eberly, J.L.; Yun, J.K.; Smith, C.D. Discovery and evaluation of inhibitors of human sphingosine kinase. *Cancer Res.* **2003**, *63*, 5962–5969. [PubMed]

13. Johnson, K.R.; Johnson, K.Y.; Crellin, H.G.; Ogretmen, B.; Boylan, A.M.; Harley, R.A.; Obeid, L.M. Immunohistochemical distribution of sphingosine kinase 1 in normal and tumor lung tissue. *J. Histochem. Cytochem.* **2005**, *53*, 1159–1166. [CrossRef] [PubMed]

14. Sobue, S.; Iwasaki, T.; Sugisaki, C.; Nagata, K.; Kikuchi, R.; Murakami, M.; Takagi, A.; Kojima, T.; Banno, Y.; Akao, Y.; et al. Quantitative rt-pcr analysis of sphingolipid metabolic enzymes in acute leukemia and myelodysplastic syndromes. *Leukemia* **2006**, *20*, 2042–2046. [CrossRef] [PubMed]

15. Kuroda, I.; Musman, M.; Ohtani, I.I.; Ichiba, T.; Tanaka, J.; Gravalos, D.G.; Higa, T. Pachastrissamine, a cytotoxic anhydrophytosphingosine from a marine sponge, *Pachastrissa* sp. *J. Nat. Prod.* **2002**, *65*, 1505–1506. [CrossRef] [PubMed]

16. Salma, Y.; Lafont, E.; Therville, N.; Carpentier, S.; Bonnafe, M.J.; Levade, T.; Genisson, Y.; Andrieu-Abadie, N. The natural marine anhydrophytosphingosine, Jaspine B, induces apoptosis in melanoma cells by interfering with ceramide metabolism. *Biochem. Pharmacol.* **2009**, *78*, 477–485. [CrossRef] [PubMed]

17. Stoica, B.A.; Movsesyan, V.A.; Lea, P.M.; Faden, A.I. Ceramide-induced neuronal apoptosis is associated with dephosphorylation of AKT, BAD, FKHR, GSK-3beta, and induction of the mitochondrial-dependent intrinsic caspase pathway. *Mol. Cell. Neurosci.* **2003**, *22*, 365–382. [CrossRef]

18. Yoo, H.; Lee, Y.S.; Lee, S.; Kim, S.; Kim, T.Y. Pachastrissamine from pachastrissa sp. Inhibits melanoma cell growth by dual inhibition of CDK2 and ERK-mediated FOXO3 downregulation. *Phytother. Res.* **2012**, *26*, 1927–1933. [CrossRef] [PubMed]

19. Lee, J.; Choi, K.; Kwon, M.; Lee, D.; Choi, M.K.; Song, I.S. Differential cytotoxic effects of Jaspine B in various cancer cells. *J. Life Sci.* **2016**, *26*, 101–109. [CrossRef]

20. Choi, M.K.; Song, I.S.; Park, S.R.; Hong, S.S.; Kim, D.D.; Chung, S.J.; Shim, C.K. Mechanism of the stationary canalicular excretion of tributylmethyl ammonium in rats with a ccl4-induced acute hepatic injury. *J. Pharm. Sci.* **2005**, *94*, 317–326. [CrossRef] [PubMed]

21. Zhang, W.; Parniak, M.A.; Sarafianos, S.G.; Empey, P.E.; Rohan, L.C. In vitro transport characteristics of efda, a novel nucleoside reverse transcriptase inhibitor using caco-2 and mdckii cell monolayers. *Eur. J. Pharmacol.* **2014**, *732*, 86–95. [CrossRef] [PubMed]

22. Choi, Y.A.; Yoon, Y.H.; Choi, K.; Kwon, M.; Goo, S.H.; Cha, J.S.; Choi, M.K.; Lee, H.S.; Song, I.S. Enhanced oral bioavailability of morin administered in mixed micelle formulation with pluronicf127 and tween80 in rats. *Biol. Pharm. Bull.* **2015**, *38*, 208–217. [CrossRef] [PubMed]

23. Oude Elferink, R.P.; Meijer, D.K.; Kuipers, F.; Jansen, P.L.; Groen, A.K.; Groothuis, G.M. Hepatobiliary secretion of organic compounds; molecular mechanisms of membrane transport. *Biochim. Biophys. Acta* **1995**, *1241*, 215–268. [CrossRef]

24. Martinez-Augustin, O.; Sanchez de Medina, F. Intestinal bile acid physiology and pathophysiology. *World J. Gastroenterol.* **2008**, *14*, 5630–5640. [CrossRef] [PubMed]

25. Song, I.S.; Choi, M.K.; Shim, W.S.; Shim, C.K. Transport of organic cationic drugs: Effect of ion-pair formation with bile salts on the biliary excretion and pharmacokinetics. *Pharmacol. Ther.* **2013**, *138*, 142–154. [CrossRef] [PubMed]

26. Song, I.S.; Chung, S.J.; Shim, C.K. Contribution of ion pair complexation with bile salts to biliary excretion of organic cations in rats. *Am. J. Physiol. Gastrointest. Liver Physiol.* **2001**, *281*, 515–525.

27. Song, I.S.; Han, Y.H.; Chung, S.J.; Shim, C.K. Contribution of ion-pair complexation with bile salts to the transport of organic cations across llc-pk1 cell monolayers. *Pharm. Res.* **2003**, *20*, 597–604. [CrossRef] [PubMed]

28. Yoshimitsu, Y.; Oishi, S.; Miyagaki, J.; Inuki, S.; Ohno, H.; Fujii, N. Pachastrissamine (Jaspine B) and its stereoisomers inhibit sphingosine kinases and atypical protein kinase c. *Bioorg. Med. Chem.* **2011**, *19*, 5402–5408. [CrossRef] [PubMed]

29. Boyer, J.L.; Scheig, R.L.; Klatskin, G. The effect of sodium taurocholate on the hepatic metabolism of sulfobromophthalein sodium (bsp). The role of bile flow. *J. Clin. Investig.* **1970**, *49*, 206–215. [CrossRef] [PubMed]

30. Yang, J.; Jamei, M.; Yeo, K.R.; Tucker, G.T.; Rostami-Hodjegan, A. Prediction of intestinal first-pass drug metabolism. *Curr. Drug Metab.* **2007**, *8*, 676–684. [CrossRef] [PubMed]

31. Dawson, P.A. Role of the intestinal bile acid transporters in bile acid and drug disposition. *Handb. Exp. Pharmacol.* **2011**, *201*, 169–203.

32. Prabagar, B.; Yoo, B.K.; Woo, J.S.; Kim, J.A.; Rhee, J.D.; Piao, M.G.; Choi, H.G.; Yong, C.S. Enhanced bioavailability of poorly water-soluble clotrimazole by inclusion with beta-cyclodextrin. *Arch. Pharm. Res.* **2007**, *30*, 249–254. [CrossRef] [PubMed]

33. Valle, J.W.; Armstrong, A.; Newman, C.; Alakhov, V.; Pietrzynski, G.; Brewer, J.; Campbell, S.; Corrie, P.; Rowinsky, E.K.; Ranson, M. A phase 2 study of sp1049c, doxorubicin in p-glycoprotein-targeting pluronics, in patients with advanced adenocarcinoma of the esophagus and gastroesophageal junction. *Investig. New Drugs* **2011**, *29*, 1029–1037. [CrossRef] [PubMed]

34. Liang, H.; Yang, Q.; Deng, L.; Lu, J.; Chen, J. Phospholipid-tween 80 mixed micelles as an intravenous delivery carrier for paclitaxel. *Drug Dev. Ind. Pharm.* **2011**, *37*, 597–605. [CrossRef] [PubMed]

35. Adedokun, O.J.; Sandborn, W.J.; Feagan, B.G.; Rutgeerts, P.; Xu, Z.; Marano, C.W.; Johanns, J.; Zhou, H.; Davis, H.M.; Cornillie, F.; et al. Association between serum concentration of infliximab and efficacy in adult patients with ulcerative colitis. *Gastroenterology* **2014**, *147*, 1296–1307. [CrossRef] [PubMed]

36. Kuo, M.T.; Chen, H.H.; Song, I.S.; Savaraj, N.; Ishikawa, T. The roles of copper transporters in cisplatin resistance. *Cancer Metastasis Rev.* **2007**, *26*, 71–83. [CrossRef] [PubMed]

37. Kwon, Y.; Song, J.; Bae, H.; Kim, W.J.; Lee, J.Y.; Han, G.H.; Lee, S.K.; Kim, S. Synthesis and biological evaluation of carbocyclic analogues of pachastrissamine. *Mar. Drugs* **2015**, *13*, 824–837. [CrossRef] [PubMed]

38. Choi, M.K.; Kwon, M.; Ahn, J.H.; Kim, N.J.; Bae, M.A.; Song, I.S. Transport characteristics and transporter-based drug-drug interactions of tm-25659, a novel taz modulator. *Biopharm. Drug Dispos.* **2014**, *35*, 183–194. [CrossRef] [PubMed]

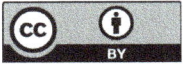

Article

Angiotensin I-Converting Enzyme (ACE) Inhibitory Activity, Antioxidant Properties, Phenolic Content and Amino Acid Profiles of *Fucus spiralis* L. Protein Hydrolysate Fractions

Lisete Paiva [1], Elisabete Lima [1,2,*], Ana Isabel Neto [3] and José Baptista [1,2]

[1]   Biotechnology Centre of Azores (CBA), University of Azores, 9501-801 Ponta Delgada, Portugal;
      lisete.s.paiva@uac.pt (L.P.); jose.ab.baptista@uac.pt (J.B.)
[2]   Research Center for Agricultural Technology (CITA-A), University of Azores,
      9501-801 Ponta Delgada, Portugal
[3]   Azorean Biodiversity Group, Centre for Ecology, Evolution and Environmental Changes (CE3C),
      Department of Biology, University of Azores, 9501-801 Ponta Delgada, Portugal; ana.im.neto@uac.pt
*   Correspondence: elisabete.mc.lima@uac.pt; Tel.: +351-296-650-182

Received: 2 September 2017; Accepted: 9 October 2017; Published: 13 October 2017

Abstract: Food protein-derived hydrolysates with multi-bioactivities such as antihypertensive and antioxidant properties have recently received special attention since both activities can play significant roles in preventing cardiovascular diseases. This study reports, for the first time, the angiotensin I-converting enzyme (ACE)-inhibition and antioxidant properties of ultrafiltrate fractions (UF) with different molecular weight ranges (<1, 1–3 and ≥3 kDa) obtained from *Fucus spiralis* protein hydrolysate (FSPH) digested with cellulase–bromelain. The amino acids profile, recovery yield, protein, peptide and total phenolic contents of these FSPH-UF, and the in vitro digestibility of *F. spiralis* crude protein were also investigated. FSPH-UF ≥3 kDa presented remarkably higher ACE-inhibition, yield, peptide and polyphenolic (phlorotannins) contents. Antioxidant analysis showed that FSPH-UF <1 kDa and ≥3 kDa exhibited significantly higher scavenging of 2,2-diphenyl-1-picrylhydrazyl radical and ferrous ion-chelating (FIC) activity. FSPH-UF ≥3 kDa had also notably higher ferric reducing antioxidant power (FRAP). Strong correlations were observed between ACE-inhibition and antioxidant activities (FIC and FRAP). The results suggest that ACE-inhibition and antioxidant properties of FSPH-UF may be due to the bioactive peptides and polyphenols released during the enzymatic hydrolysis. In conclusion, this study shows the potential use of defined size FSPH-UF for the prevention/treatment of hypertension and/or oxidative stress-related diseases.

Keywords: edible brown algae; protein enzymatic hydrolysate; ultrafiltration; ACE-inhibition; antioxidant properties; phlorotannins; peptide fractions; amino acids composition; marine functional foods; cardiovascular-health

---

1. Introduction

Marine organisms, including macro-algae, are a valuable source of structurally diverse bioactive metabolites with various biological activities due to their living mode in highly competitive and aggressive surroundings, which are very different in many aspects from terrestrial environment, a situation that demands the production of quite specific and potent bioactive molecules. As a result, the importance of these organisms as a natural resource of bioactive compounds, which may lead to the development of new drugs and functional foods or nutraceuticals, is growing rapidly [1].

Macro-algae have been consumed in Asian countries since ancient times and their dietary intake has been shown to decrease blood pressure in humans [2]. However, the angiotensin

I-converting enzyme (ACE) inhibitory activity from macro-algae has not been extensively studied [3]. ACE belongs to the class of zinc metal proteases that catalyzes the conversion of angiotensin I to a potent vasoconstrictor angiotensin II and also promotes the degradation of the vasodilator bradykinin [4]. Therefore, this multifunctional enzyme plays a key role in the control of blood pressure, since the inhibition of its activity leads to a decrease in the angiotensin II concentration and an increase in the bradykinin level, and consequently in the reduction of hypertension that is one of the major causes of chronic diseases and a high risk factor of cardiovascular diseases worldwide [5]. A wide variety of synthetic drugs have been extensively used in treatment of hypertension and most of them have an ACE-inhibitory activity, however, these drugs can cause certain adverse side effects [6]. Therefore, searching for ACE-inhibitors from natural resources, such as marine organisms including macro-algae [3,7–9], has shown a growing interest in the field of nutraceutical, pharmaceutical and functional foods industries. The most commonly studied natural ACE-inhibitors were protein hydrolysates and peptides, however, others molecules that affect the ACE activity include the phorotannins group that are the predominant polyphenols in brown algae, being particularly abundant in Fucaceae [10–13]. In addition to its strong ACE-inhibition, phlorotannins have been recently demonstrated to possess numerous health benefits, including potent antioxidant effects (for a review see [14]). Since functional food products with multi-bioactivities are receiving wider attention, the potential antioxidant of macro-algal protein hydrolysates/peptides with ACE-inhibitory activity has also been investigated [15–17]. In fact, it is well known that natural antioxidants are powerful substances that play an important role against various diseases (atherosclerosis, cancer, chronic inflammation, cardiovascular disorders, hypertension) and ageing process, directly related to oxidative stress [18].

There is substantial scientific evidence that enzymatic hydrolysis of food protein sources is an efficient method to recover potent bioactive peptides that may present lower side effects [1,19]. Furthermore, enzymatic proteolysis can also release other bioactive compounds such as phorotannins bound to proteins, as reported for some brown macro-algae [20].

The Azores Islands (Portugal) being isolated in the middle of Atlantic Ocean and surrounded by waters with low pollution levels [21] is a very promising location to look for new marine ingredients with medicine-like effects in treating or preventing chronic diseases. Traditionally, the Azorean population has gathered seaweeds either as food or for chemicals extraction. The brown seaweed *Fucus spiralis*, which is abundant in the Azorean intertidal zone, is a local delicacy, particularly the frond tips (the receptacles) that are picked and eaten fresh [22]. Previous studies on its nutritional and/or pharmacological value from our research group have reported that *F. spiralis* is a good source of valuable biochemical compounds [23] and its methanol extract could also be a source of powerful ACE-inhibitory phlorotannins with potential impact on human health [9]. *F. spiralis* from other origins have been also demonstrated to possess high antioxidant properties, mainly linked to its phlorotannin content [24–26].

This is, for the best of our knowledge, the first study of *F. spiralis* enzymatic protein hydrolysate as source of compounds with multi-bioactivities for potential use in food and pharmaceutical industries and it was aimed to: (i) optimize the protein extraction process to obtain higher yield of *F. spiralis* protein hydrolysate, (ii) fractionate the cellulase–bromelain protein hydrolysate by ultrafiltration membranes into different molecular weight fractions (<1, 1–3 and ≥3 kDa), (iii) evaluate the ultrafiltrate fractions for multifunctional properties in vitro, namely the ACE-inhibitory activity and the antioxidant properties using different assays, such as the scavenging of 2,2-diphenyl-1-picrylhydrazyl radical, the ferrous ion-chelating and the ferric reducing antioxidant power, (iv) determine the amino acids profile, recovery yield, protein, peptide and total phenolic contents of the ultrafiltrate fractions, and (v) evaluate the in vitro digestibility of *F. spiralis* crude protein. The findings of the current study can also contribute to the increasing database of medicinal macro-algae.

2. Results and Discussion

2.1. F. spiralis Protein Content and In Vitro Protein Digestibility Evaluation

Results revealed that *F. spiralis* has a protein content of 8.53 ± 0.03% (on a dry basis), which is within the range reported for brown algae (3.0–15.0%) [27]. *F. spiralis* protein digestibility, expressed as a relative percentage of sodium caseinate digestibility normalized at 100%, was 85.95 ± 0.85%. It is well known that amino acid profiles are important in evaluating the proteins quality, and their digestibility is the primary determinant of its amino acid availability, but the in vivo algae protein digestibility is still poorly described. However, the high protein digestibility determined in vitro suggests that *F. spiralis* can be used as a complementary source of food proteins for human and animal nutrition, which according to Fleurence [27], would be a promising way for the exploitation of marine resources in Europe.

2.2. Preparation of F. spiralis Protein Hydrolysate (FSPH) and Its Fractionation by Ultrafiltration

In this study, *F. spiralis* protein concentrate after a two steps hydrolysis with a combination of two enzymes (cellulase and bromelain) followed by membrane ultrafiltration yielded three fractions ($Fr_1 < 1$ kDa, 1 kDa $\leq Fr_2 < 3$ kDa and $Fr_3 \geq 3$ kDa) that presented values of 206.28, 53.72 and 703.95 mg/g of dry FSPH, respectively (Table 1). These fractions were assessed for their ACE-inhibitory and antioxidant activities in order to find new marine sources of functional food products with multi-bioactivities for application in food and medicine industries. Indeed, according to some researchers [17,20], enzymatic hydrolysis can enhance the release of ACE inhibitory and antioxidant compounds (such as peptides and polyphenols) from the algal matrix. On the other hand, the use of carbohydrases, such as cellulase that breakdown cellulose and some related polysaccharides [28], can be useful before proteolytic enzymes applications. In fact the results showed that, when cellulase was used before the enzymatic hydrolysis with bromelain, the yield of *F. spiralis* protein concentrate was 1.5-fold increased. The choice of bromelain was based on our previous study [29] that showed the higher proteolytic activity (number of peptides) of bromelain as compared to the other nine commercial proteases tested using *F. spiralis* water extracts.

Table 1. Angiotensin I-converting enzyme (ACE) inhibitory activity, recovery yield, protein and peptide contents of *F. spiralis* protein hydrolysate (FSPH) fractions obtained by ultrafiltration.

Sample	Yield (mg/g of DW FSPH)	ACE-Inhibition		Protein Content (mg/g of DW FSPH)	Peptide Content (mg/g of DW FSPH)
		Percentage	IC$_{50}$ Value (mg/mL)		
$Fr_1 < 1$ kDa	206.28	45.08 ± 0.66 [a]	1.850 ± 0.06 [b]	123.15 ± 2.78 [a]	43.81 ± 2.27 [a]
1 kDa $\leq Fr_2 < 3$ kDa	53.72	41.93 ± 1.62 [a]	2.000 ± 0.06 [b]	336.28 ± 4.96 [b]	35.91 ± 1.58 [a]
$Fr_3 \geq 3$ kDa	703.95	86.85 ± 1.89 [b]	0.500 ± 0.03 [a]	474.03 ± 4.44 [b]	243.82 ± 2.9 [b]

Values are mean ± SD ($n = 3$). Different superscript letters are significantly different ($p < 0.05$). IC$_{50}$ value defined as the concentration which inhibits 50% of the ACE activity (tested concentration = 2 mg/mL). Captopril, used as a positive control for ACE-inhibition, showed an IC$_{50}$ value of 0.163 ng/mL. DW, dry weight.

A two-steps hydrolysis was been previously used by our research group on other macro-algae proteins, to promote the release of low-MW (molecular weight) peptides [3]. Furthermore, this previous report also revealed that bromelain exhibited the highest specificity in the generation of ACE-inhibitory peptides from *Ulva rigida* protein. Other studies on other marine resources, such as different kinds of fish, also showed that bromelain is the most efficient protease tested for the production of protein hydrolysates with higher bioactivities (ACE-inhibitory and/or antioxidant activities) [30–32]. On the other hand, a molecular weight cut-off (MWCO) dialysis of FSPH was further used as means of enhancing its bioactivities, as well as to provide insights into the molecular weight distribution of the bioactive compounds presented in the hydrolysate. Furthermore, it should also be pointed out that the use of bioactive MWCO fractions instead of its purified active constituents for the development of functional foods presents multiple advantages. In fact, besides its low cost production and high production yield, MWCO fractions are formed by sets of compounds which could exhibit different biological activities and may act in synergy to increase its physiological effects on the organism [33]. In addition, the incorporation of protein hydrolysate fractions to foods could confer low cost desirable nutritional and functional properties.

2.3. Protein and Peptide Contents of FSPH Fractions

Protein and peptide contents of FSPH ultrafiltration fractions are also shown in Table 1, being the higher values in Fr_3 (474.03 ± 4.44 and 243.82 ± 2.91 mg/g of dry FSPH, respectively). The Fr_1 and Fr_2 presented also a higher value of protein (123.15 ± 2.78 and 336.28 ± 4.96 mg/g of dry FSPH, respectively), but only a small content of peptides (43.81 ± 2.27 and 35.91 ± 1.58 mg/g of dry FSPH, respectively) as compared to Fr_3.

2.4. Amino Acids Composition of FSPH Fractions

It is known that food protein hydrolysate/fractions containing appropriate amounts of amino acids with strong contribution properties could be potential candidates for use as potent antihypertensive and antioxidant agents [34]. As shown in Table 2, the amino acid's profiles varied among the FSPH ultrafiltration fractions in terms of individual and total amino acid contents. The total amino acid content in Fr_3 was 562.75 mg/g of dry FSPH which is significantly higher than those found in Fr_1 and Fr_2 (196.28 mg/g and 242.48 mg/g of dry FSPH, respectively). All the FSPH fractions showed remarkably higher percentage of the hydrophobic amino acids group (65.4–90.1% of the total amino acids), being valine the major amino acid in all fractions with 79.2%, 86.3% and 42.1% of the total amino acids in Fr_1, Fr_2 and Fr_3, respectively. Glutamic acid, tyrosine, aspartic acid and isoleucine were the other major amino acids in Fr_3, representing 8.2%, 6.8%, 6.7% and 5.8% of the total amino acids, respectively. In fractions Fr_1 and Fr_2, lysine and glutamic acid were the other major amino acids present. The amino acids content of Fr_1 was very similar to that of Fr_2. Overall, the Fr_3 had the highest concentration of aromatic amino acids as well as hydrophobic aliphatic amino acids such as isoleucine, leucine, alanine, methionine and proline that, according to the previous reports [17,33,34], may promote the ACE-inhibitory and antioxidant activities of food protein hydrolysates/fractions.

According to the literature, most seaweeds contains all essential amino acids and some also present high levels of acidic amino acids (8.0–44.0% on a dry basis) and low levels of histidine, threonine, tryptophan, lysine, methionine and cysteine [35]. In our study methionine, threonine and lysine, in which many cereals are deficient [36], were presented in reasonable percentages, particularly in Fr_3 and in Fr_1.

2.5. Total Phenolic Content (TPC) of FSPH Fractions

The TPC was quantified as phloroglucinol equivalents (PE), and the results (Figure 1) revealed that Fr_3 was the one with remarkably higher values (106.83 ± 0.76 mg PE/g of DW) followed by Fr_2 and Fr_1 with the values of 53.17 ± 0.76 and 15.00 ± 0.50 mg PE/g of DW, respectively, suggesting that high-MW phlorotannins are the largest pool of phenolic compounds in *F. spiralis*. On the other hand, the same order was observed for the protein content of FSPH fractions, as previously mentioned, suggesting that the fraction having a high content of protein tended to have a higher TPC. These findings are in accordance with Athukorala and Jeon [37] for the Flavourzyme *Ecklonia cava* hydrolysate fractions.

The TPC values of *F. spiralis* in the present study were higher than the ones reported by Tierney et al. [38] for Irish *F. spiralis*. This fact may be related with differences in the extraction methodology employed. Furthermore, significant intra-species variations of TPC in brown fucoid algae are well documented, showing the effect of several factors such as algae size, age, tissue type and environmental factors, including nutrient availability, light intensity, ultraviolet radiation, salinity, water depth and season [14,39].

Table 2. Amino acid profiles of *F. spiralis* protein hydrolysate fractions (mg amino acids/g of DW FSPH) obtained by ultrafiltration.

Amino Acid (AA)	*F. spiralis* Protein Hydrolysate (FSPH) Fraction		
	Fr$_1$ < 1 kDa	1 kDa ≤ Fr$_2$ < 3 kDa	Fr$_3$ ≥ 3 kDa
Alanine	tc	tc	25.34 ± 0.13
Glycine	tc	tc	22.38 ± 0.13
Valine	155.53 ± 2.25	209.37 ± 3.35	236.83 ± 4.65
Threonine	1.22 ± 0.08	1.71 ± 0.03	17.42 ± 0.13
Serine	2.75 ± 0.06	3.18 ± 0.03	19.36 ± 0.16
Leucine	2.24 ± 0.12	2.85 ± 0.05	25.35 ± 0.17
Isoleucine	1.89 ± 0.03	2.84 ± 0.06	32.55 ± 0.43
Proline	1.34 ± 0.05	1.93 ± 0.03	12.47 ± 0.11
Methionine	tc	tc	20.07 ± 0.31
Aspartic acid	3.63 ± 0.07	4.53 ± 0.10	37.53 ± 0.35
Phenylalanine	1.80 ± 0.02	1.49 ± 0.02	15.13 ± 0.15
Glutamic acid	10.40 ± 0.10	7.01 ± 0.22	46.33 ± 0.42
Lysine	15.48 ± 0.20	7.57 ± 0.11	13.82 ± 0.13
Tyrosine	tc	tc	38.17 ± 0.21
Arginine	tc	tc	tc
Histidine	tc	tc	tc
Tryptophan	ND	ND	ND
Total AA	196.28 [a]	242.48 [a]	562.75 [b]
AA distribution (%)			
Hydrophobic	82.94 [a]	90.10 [a]	65.35 [b]
Hydrophilic	15. 04 [a]	7.88 [b]	17.36 [a]
Neutral	2.02 [b]	2.02 [b]	17.29 [a]
Aromatic	0.92 [b]	0.61 [b]	9.47 [a]
Branched-side chains	81.34 [a]	88.69 [a]	52.37 [b]
Negatively charged	7.15 [b]	4.76 [c]	14.90 [a]
Positively charged	7.89 [a]	3.12 [b]	2.46 [b]

Values are mean ± SD (*n* = 3). Means with different superscripts letters in the same row differ significantly (*p* < 0.05). Hydrophobic AA (Ala, Val, Leu, Ile, Pro, Met, Phe). Hydrophilic AA (Asp, Glu, Lys, Arg, His). Neutral AA (Gly, Thr, Ser, Tyr). Aromatic AA (Phe, Tyr). Branched-side chains AA (Val, Leu, Ile). Negatively charged AA (Asp, Glu). Positively charged AA (Lys, Arg, His). Tryptophan is not detected in this methodology. DW, dry weight; ND, not detected; tc, traces.

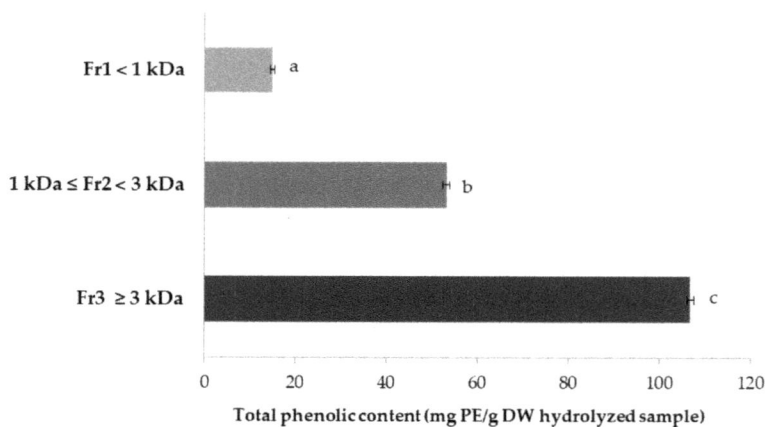

Figure 1. Total phenolic contents (TPC) of *F. spiralis* protein hydrolysate fractions obtained by ultrafiltration (tested concentration 2 mg/mL). Values are mean ± SD (*n* = 3). Different letters are significantly different (*p* < 0.05). Legend: DW, dry weight; PE, phloroglucinol equivalents.

According to the literature, brown macro-algae are a well-known source of phlorotannins, a structurally unique polyphenols that have gathered much attention due to their numerous bioactivities with high commercial interest for pharmaceutical, nutraceutical, cosmetic and especially food industries. Phlorotannins, which have been reported as the only phenolic group detected in some brown algae, such as *Fucus vesiculosus* [14], are highly hydrophilic components with a wide range of molecular sizes ranging between 126 Da and 650 kDa, although they are more commonly found in the 10 to 100 kDa range, particularly in the Fucaceae family [11,25]. Only few reports have focused on phlorotannin profile from *Fucus* spp. Phlorotannins with high degree of polymerization were observed in *F. spiralis* from Canada [40]; this information is important because it is known that ACE-inhibitory and antioxidant activities may depend on the degree of polymerization of phlorotannin derivatives [11,25]. Furthermore, sparse characterization of individual phlorotannin components has been carried out in *F. spiralis* species [9,24,41].

2.6. ACE-Inhibitory Activity of FSPH Fractions

The ACE-inhibition was determined by HPLC-UV method and the results (Table 1) revealed a remarkably higher activity in Fr_3 followed by Fr_1 and Fr_2 with percentage values of 86.85 ± 1.89%, 45.08 ± 0.66% and 41.93 ± 1.62% and IC_{50} values of 0.500 ± 0.03, 1.850 ± 0.06 and 2.000 ± 0.06 mg/mL, respectively. However, all FSPH fractions showed higher IC_{50} values as compared to captopril (0.163 ng/mL), a synthetic ACE-inhibitor used in this study as a positive control. A comparison of the present data with other results is quite difficult due to the lack of literature on ACE-inhibition of *Fucus* spp. protein hydrolysates/fractions, as well as variations in hydrolysis conditions. However, the ACE IC_{50} values obtained in this study (0.500–2.000 mg/mL) were similar to those reported for bromelain–alcalase protein hydrolysate fractions from the sea cucumber *Acaudina molpadioidea* (0.615–1.975 mg/mL) [42]. Furthermore, our values were similar or lower than those described for *Porphyra yezoensis* hydrolysates (1.520–3.210 mg/mL) [7], and are within the range reported for enzymatic hydrolysates from different protein sources (0.20–2.47 mg/mL) with antihypertensive activity in spontaneously hypertensive rats [43].

The difference in the ACE-inhibition among hydrolysate fractions could be related to the differences in amino acid compositions (Table 2) and their sequences, as well as the peptide sizes. Indeed, ACE-inhibitory peptides are usually between 2 and 30 amino acids in size [44]. On the other hand, according to the literature [17,45,46], the presence of aromatic and branched-side chain amino acids (BCAA) in peptides may promote the ACE-inhibition of food protein hydrolysates/fractions. Thus, the results of this study suggested that the relatively good ACE-inhibition (over 40%) of the low-MW FSPH fractions (Fr_1 and Fr_2) can be attributed to the presence of low-MW peptides plus the highest concentration of BCAA. In turn, the Fr_3 was the one with significantly higher aromatic amino acids content that make a substantial contribution to its ACE-inhibition by blocking angiotensin II production, probably due to their high steric properties and low lipophilicity [45]. Furthermore, the remarkably higher ACE-inhibition of Fr_3 could also be due to the contribution of polyphenols (phlorotannins) released during the enzymatic hydrolysis and concentrated in this fraction. In fact, some reports indicate that brown algae might have strong ACE-like inhibitors associated not only with peptides but also with phlorotannins [11,12]. Wijesinghe et al. [12] also reported that the ACE-inhibition may be closely associated with protein-binding abilities of phlorotannins, which are characteristic of all tannins. Indeed, it has been well described that tannins have the ability to form strong complexes with proteins, either reversibly by hydrogen bonding through peptide or amide linkages or irreversibly by covalent condensation, and that polyphenolic compounds inhibit ACE activity through sequestration of the enzyme metal factor (Zn^{2+}) [47]. A previous study by our research group [9] already reported that the strong ACE-inhibition by Azorean *F. spiralis* methanol extract may be due to its rich content of high-MW phorotannins, also concentrated in the MWCO ≥3 kDa fraction. Thus, *F. spiralis* phorotannins could be considered as potential phytopharmaceuticals for the development of new ACE inhibitors. On the other hand, it should be also pointed out that for food industry, enzymatic extracts, as obtained in the present study, is safer for consumers than organic solvent extracts, since the enzymatic method does not utilizes any organic solvent or other toxic chemicals.

2.7. Antioxidant Activities of FSPH Fractions

2.7.1. 2,2-Diphenyl-1-picrylhydrazyl (DPPH) Free Radical Scavenging Activity (FRSA) Assay

The scavenging activity of DPPH free radicals had been used extensively to determine the antioxidant power of bioactive natural products. The results revealed that FRSA increased with increasing FSPH fraction concentration (Figure 2). At the highest concentration of 200 μg/mL the Fr_1 presented the highest FRSA value (86.03 ± 0.25%), followed by Fr_3 (80.50 ± 0.53%) whereas the Fr_2 presented the lowest value (32.73 ± 0.32%); furthermore, the FRSA of Fr_1 was comparable to that of the commercial antioxidant butylated hydroxytoluene (BHT). Tierney et al. [38] reported a lower value (6.18 ± 2.16%, the reciprocal of the IC_{50}) of FRSA for the fraction with a MW of 3 kDa obtained from Irish *F. spiralis* hydrolysate digested with carbohydrase Viscozyme. These results may suggest that the enzymatic method used in the present study was more effective for the generation of antioxidant hydrolysates from *F. spiralis*. Several studies have also shown that, generally, low-MW hydrolysate fractions have higher DPPH radical scavenging activity than in high-MW hydrolysate fractions [48,49]. However, Fr_3 showed an IC_{50} value of 55 μg/mL that is lower than Fr_1 (85 μg/mL). Similar results were reported by Udenigwe et al. [50], who found that the high-MW fractions of flaxseed protein hydrolysate showed better FRSA as compared to the low-MW fractions.

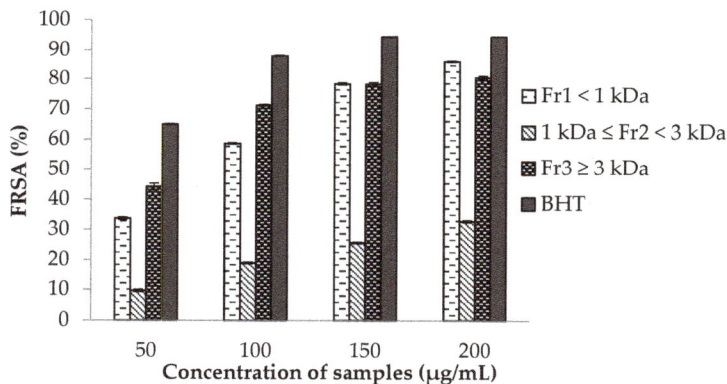

Figure 2. Free radical scavenging activity (FRSA) of *F. spiralis* protein hydrolysate fractions obtained by ultrafiltration. BHT (butylated hydroxytoluene) was used as positive control. Values are mean ± SD (*n* = 3).

The difference in the FRSA among the hydrolysate fractions might be related not only to their different peptide sizes but also to the differences in the amino acid compositions (Table 2) and their sequences, as well as the synergistic contributions of the active compounds. Indeed, research by Chen et al. [51] and Guo et al. [52] has demonstrated that DPPH radical scavenging activity is related to the amino acids composition. It was reported that aromatic amino acids and hydrophobic aliphatic amino acids (such as alanine, leucine, methionine and valine) play an important role in the DPPH radical scavenging activity [53,54]. Alemán et al. [55] also reports that the presence of those amino acids in a peptide sequence might increase the ability to access and neutralize the reactive free radicals and consequently to enhance the antioxidant activity. In addition, acidic amino acids had showed strong positive effects on scavenging of DPPH and, in contrast, positively-charged amino acids strongly contributed negatively to FRSA [34]. Thus, the lower FRSA IC_{50} value in Fr_3 might be related to the highest content of aromatic, acidic and hydrophobic aliphatic amino acid residues, with exception for valine, as well as to the lowest positively-charged amino acids content. However, the superior TPC of Fr_3 than in low-MW fractions (Fr_1 and Fr_2), as previously mentioned, may suggest that high-MW phlorotannins are the principal contributor to the lower FRSA IC_{50} value observed. Similar results were reported by other researchers, who found that high-MWCO fractions of *Fucus* species, such as *F. vesiculosus* [39] and *F. serrata* [56], had the highest FRSA and phenolic content (phlorotannins). It should also be highlighted that a recent study [26] revealed that phlorotannin-enriched fractions from *F. spiralis* from Peniche (Portugal) have the capacity to inhibit in vitro human cellular damage promoted by reactive oxygen species. Kim et al. [57] also reported that the fraction >30 kDa of the Celluclast enzymatic extract from brown algae *Ecklonia cava* possesses high protective effects against hydrogen peroxide-induced cell damage, attributed to the presence of phlorotannins. As in the present study, this *E. cava* fraction revealed the highest TPC, whereas the lowest content was shown by the fraction <1 kDa.

2.7.2. Ferrous Ion-Chelating (FIC) Activity Assay

Since metal chelating capacity is claimed as one of the important mechanisms of antioxidant activity [58], FIC assay was also chosen to better characterize the antioxidant activity of FSPH fractions. As shown in Figure 3, and in accordance with FRSA results, Fr_3 presented the highest FIC activity ($47.33 \pm 1.15\%$) followed by Fr_1 ($40.28 \pm 1.21\%$), and Fr_2 the lowest value ($28.47 \pm 1.21\%$), but no significant difference was observed between Fr_1 and Fr_3. Similar results were found by Tierney et al. [38] for FIC activity ($50.67 \pm 5.58\%$) in the fraction with MW of 3 kDa from Irish *F. spiralis* Viscozyme hydrolysate. The FSPH Fr_1 and Fr_3 were moderate metal chelating agents as compared to the synthetic antioxidant EDTA, a potent metal-ion chelator used in this study as a positive control.

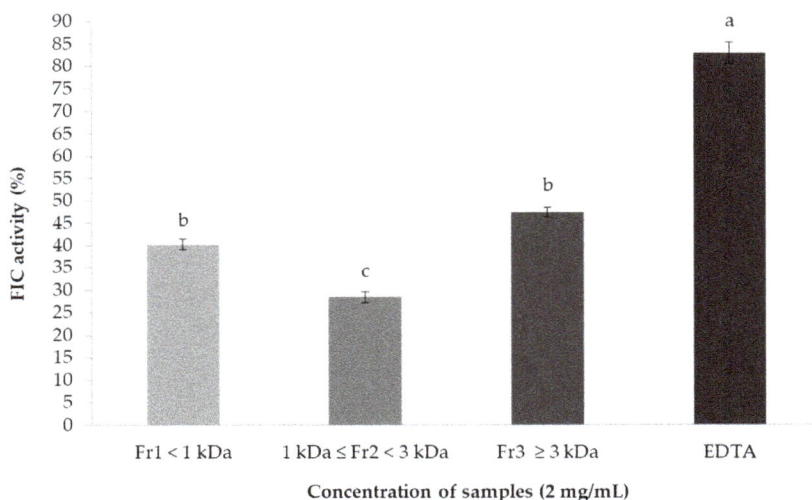

Figure 3. Ferrous ion-chelating (FIC) activities of *F. spiralis* protein hydrolysate fractions obtained by ultrafiltration. EDTA (ethylenediaminetetraacetic acid) was used as positive control. Values are mean $\pm$ SD ($n = 3$). Different letters are significantly different ($p < 0.05$).

Most of the reported peptides exhibiting chelating activities were those with low-MW [59], which explains the FIC activity of the lower-MW Fr_1. However, higher FIC activity in some other food hydrolysate fractions is linked to a larger peptide size [60]. Furthermore, peptides with high chelating activities have a high content of acidic amino acids [17]. As shown in Table 2, the Fr_3

had the highest content of negatively charged amino acids followed by Fr_1. On the other hand, Fr_3 presented the highest TPC value, as previously mentioned. Thus, the highest FIC activity of the higher-MW Fr_3 can be attributed to larger size bioactive compounds, such as the large peptides and the high-MW phlorotannins, released during the enzymatic hydrolysis and concentrated in this fraction. Indeed, some studies have demonstrated that polyphenols derived from algae are potent ferrous-ion chelators [61] and that its metal chelating potency is dependent upon their unique phenolic structure and the number and location of the hydroxyl groups [62]. However, to better evaluate the contribution of the polyphenols to the FIC activity of *F. spiralis*, additional research is needed on structural information of the bioactive compounds.

2.7.3. Ferric Reducing Antioxidant Power (FRAP) Assay

The highest FRAP was observed in Fr_3 followed by Fr_1 and Fr_2 fractions (Figure 4) for the higher concentration used (28.41 µg/mL), presenting absorbance values of 0.538, 0.334 and 0.185, respectively. The presence of reducers (antioxidants) causes the conversion of the Fe^{3+}/ferricyanide complex used in this method to the ferrous form. Therefore, by measuring the formation of Perl's Prussian blue at 700 nm, we can monitor the Fe^{2+} concentration, that indicates a higher reducing power, compared to that of BHT, which is known to be a strong reducing agent. The information on FRAP activity is important because the reducing capacity of a compound/fraction may serve as a significant indicator of reductones, that are reported to be terminators of free radicals chain reaction, presents in the samples [63–65].

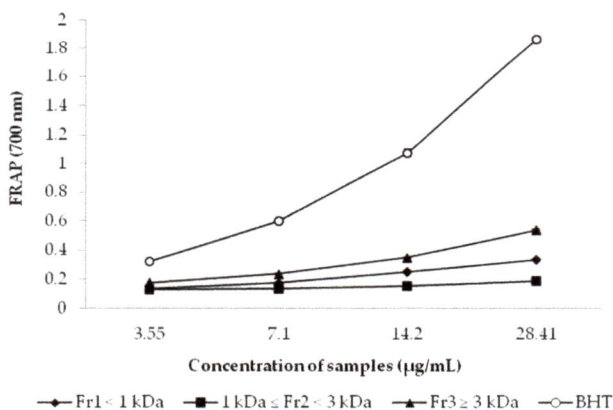

Figure 4. Ferric reducing antioxidant power (FRAP) of *F. spiralis* protein hydrolysate fractions obtained by ultrafiltration. BHT (butylated hydroxytoluene) was used as positive control. Values are mean ± SD ($n = 3$).

In accordance to the outlined for FRSA and FIC activity results, the highest FRAP of Fr_3 may be due, mainly, to its rich content of high-MW phlorotannins. Our findings are in agreement with previous studies on FRAP of MW-fractionated hydrolysates/extracts from other algae samples, such as the Irish *F. spiralis* [25,38] and other *Fucus* species (*F. vesiculosus* and *F. serrata*) [39,56]. Furthermore, as shown in Table 2, Fr_3 presented the highest content of the amino acids glutamic acid, aspartic acid, glycine, methionine and threonine as well as lysine in lower amount that, based on Udenigwe and Aluko [34], is a type of pattern that could have contributed to the highest FRAP observed in this FSPH fraction. Moreover, other authors observed that higher FRAP in some other food hydrolysate fractions is also linked to a larger size peptide content [60], that is in agreement with our results.

2.8. Pearson Correlation between Parameters

A significant correlation was found to occur among the methods for the antioxidant activities determination in all FSPH fractions (Table 3). FRSA and FIC activity ($r = 0.890$) were strongly correlated as well as FIC activity and FRAP ($r = 0.973$). A moderate correlation was found between FRSA and FRAP ($r = 0.760$). Concerning the correlation between TPC and antioxidant activities, a very weak correlation exists between TPC and FRSA ($r = 0.003$), and a weak correlation between TPC and FIC activity ($r = 0.458$), however, TPC and FRAP were moderately correlated ($r = 0.652$). On the other hand, strong correlations were observed between peptide content and FIC activity or FRAP or TPC ($r = 0.805$, $r = 0.921$ and $r = 0.896$), while the correlation between peptide content and FRSA was weak ($r = 0.446$). These results may reveal that other bioactive compounds such as peptides, in addition to polyphenols (phlorotannins), are contributing to the antioxidant activities of FSPH fractions evaluated by FRSA, FIC activity and FRAP assays. Previous research by Zubia et al. [66] and Vinayak et al. [67] also reported weak correlations ($r = -0.399$ and $r = 0.397$, respectively) between TPC and FRSA of macro-algal extracts. However, it should be noted that individual polyphenols may have a considerable antioxidant potential, but there may be antagonistic or synergistic interactions between phenolic and non-phenolic compounds that may affect the bioactivity [68]. Concerning the FIC activity, the correlations observed in the present study may suggest that polyphenols (phlorotannins) are not the principal chelators in some of FSPH fractions and that others compounds such as peptides, which are also recognized as effective chelating agents [69], may be the main contributors to the observed activities. Research by Wang et al. [48,58] has reported the absence of clear correlations between TPC and FIC ability of macro-algal extracts.

Table 3. Correlation matrix of the studied parameters (Pearson correlations coefficients).

	FRSA	FIC Activity	FRAP	Total Phenolic	ACE-Inhibition	Peptide Content
FRSA	1	-	-	-	-	-
FIC activity	0.890	1		-	-	-
FRAP	0.760	0.973	1		-	-
Total phenolic	0.003	0.458	0.652	1	-	-
ACE-inhibition	0.660	0.822	0.932	0.883	1	-
Peptide content	0.446	0.805	0.921	0.896	1	1

FRSA, free radical scavenging activity; FIC, ferrous ions (Fe^{2+}) chelating; FRAP, ferric reducing antioxidant power; ACE, angiotensin I-converting enzyme.

As for ACE-inhibitory activity, a perfect correlation was observed between ACE-inhibition and peptide content ($r = 1$) and strong correlations were observed between ACE-inhibition and FIC activity ($r = 0.822$), between ACE-inhibition and FRAP ($r = 0.932$), and between ACE-inhibition and TPC ($r = 0.883$). Only the correlation between ACE-inhibition and FRSA was moderate ($r = 0.660$). These findings suggest that either some peptides, which are recognized as effective ACE-inhibitors agents or polyphenols are contributing to the ACE-inhibition observed in all FSPH fractions.

Overall results from this study suggest that ACE-inhibition and antioxidant activities observed in FSPH fractions may be due to the sum of the activities of produced peptides and released polyphenols. However, in order to better understand the contribution of peptides and polyphenols to the aforementioned bifunctional properties, a complete chemical characterization of FSPH fractions should be done in future.

3. Materials and Methods

3.1. Chemicals and Reagents

Methanol (MeOH) and acetonitrile (ACN) HPLC grade were purchased from Fluka Chemika (Steinheim, Switzerland). Ammonium sulphate, sodium carbonate (Na_2CO_3), sodium phosphate, sodium tetraborate decahydrate, iron (II) chloride, sodium hydroxide (NaOH), ethanol, phenol and

85% phosphoric acid were from E. Merck (Darmstadt, Germany). Acetyl chloride and isobutanol were purchased from Alltech Associates (Deerfield, IL, USA). Amino acids standard mixture and sequanal grade 6 N HCl were purchased from Pierce Chemicals (Rockford, IL, USA). Sodium chloride (NaCl), ethyl acetate, heptafluorobutyric anhydride (HFB-IBA), sodium caseinate, 2-mercaptoethanol, brilliant Blue G-250, albumin from bovine serum (BSA), potassium ferricyanide, iron (III) chloride, ferrozine, trichloroacetic acid (TCA), trizma base, zinc chloride, hippuric acid (HA), hippuryl-L-histidyl-L-leucine (HHL), Folin–Ciocalteu reagent (FCR), phloroglucinol, butylated hydroxytoluene (BHT), ethylenediaminetetraacetic acid (EDTA), 2,2-diphenyl-1-picrylhydrazyl (DPPH), hydrochloric acid (HCl), glutathione, *O*-phthaldialdehyde (OPA), β-mercaptoethanol, sodium dodecyl sulphate, angiotensin I-converting enzyme (ACE) from porcine kidney, bromelain (B4882), cellulase from *Aspergillus niger* (C1184), chymotrypsin (C9381), peptidase (P7500) and trypsin (T8003) were obtained from Sigma-Aldrich (St. Louis, MO, USA). Ultrafiltration membrane system and membranes were purchased from Millipore Co (Bedford, MA, USA).

3.2. Collection and Preparation of F. spiralis Sample

F. spiralis Linnaeus (Ochrophyta, Phaeophyceae) sample was collected in January 2013 from the littoral of São Miguel Island of Azores Archipelago (37°40′ N and 25°31′ W), Portugal, and a voucher specimen was prepared (voucher number AZB, SMG-13-04) and deposited in the Herbarium AZB—Ruy Telles Palhinha of the Department of Biology at the University of Azores. Within 24 h of collection, *F. spiralis* sample was first washed in seawater followed by distilled water to remove encrusting material, epiphytes and salts, and then air-dried and stored in an air-tight container in a freezer ($-80\,°C$) for not more than 6 months until further analysis. Prior to the analytical procedures, the sample was defrosted and dried at 40–45 °C for 48 h (avoiding overheating that could lead to oxidation), and then was grounded into a fine powder of 0.5 mm particle size, re-dried at 40 °C and stored in the dark under N_2 in a desiccator at a refrigerated temperature of 4–5 °C.

3.3. Extraction of Protein from F. spiralis

The protein of *F. spiralis* was extracted according to the method described by Wong et al. [70] with slight modifications. Five grams of sample powder were suspended in deionized water (1:10 *w/v*) to induce cell lysis by osmotic shock that facilitated subsequent protein extraction. The suspension was gently stirred overnight at 35 °C, which was found to be the optimal temperature for macro-algae protein solubility. After incubation, the suspension was centrifuged at $10,000\times g$ and 4 °C for 20 min. The supernatant was collected and the pellet was re-suspended in deionized water with 0.5% 2-mercaptoethanol (*v/v*) being the pH adjusted to 12.0 with 1 M NaOH. The solution was gently stirred at room temperature for 2 h before centrifugation under the same conditions as above. The second supernatant was collected and combined with the first one. The combined supernatant was stirred at 4 °C and the pH was adjusted to 7.0 before precipitation with ammonium sulphate. The extraction method mentioned above was repeated three times on the residue. The combined supernatant was precipitated by slowly adding ammonium sulphate, with stirring, until 85% saturation (60 g/100 mL) and allowed to stand for 30 min. Then the solution (precipitated protein) was removed by centrifugation at $10,000\times g$, 4 °C for 20 min. The pellet obtained was dialyzed against distilled water until the total dissolved solutes of dialysate, measured by its conductivity, was similar to that of the distilled water. The retentate containing the protein concentrate of *F. spiralis* was lyophilized in a freeze-drier and stored at $-20\,°C$ until required. The protein content was determined by Bradford method [71] using BSA as the calibration standard.

3.4. In Vitro F. spiralis Protein Digestibility Evaluation

The in vitro digestibility of *F. spiralis* protein concentrate suspension was determined using a freshly prepared multiproteolytic enzyme solution (trypsin, chymotrypsin and peptidase), according to Paiva et al. [72], in order to reproduce the actual digestion environment in vivo. Fifty milliliters of aqueous protein suspension (6.25 mg protein/mL) in glass distilled water were adjusted to pH 8.0, while stirring in a 37 °C water bath. The multi-enzyme solution [1.6 mg/mL trypsin (10,000 BAEE units/mg protein), 3.1 mg/mL chymotrypsin (80 units/mg solid) and 1.3 mg peptidase/mL (50–100 units/g solid)] was maintained in an ice bath and adjusted to pH 8.0. Five milliliters of the multi-enzyme solution were then added to the protein suspension and the pH change in the mixture, caused by the enzymatic digestion, was measured after exactly 10 min. Sodium caseinate was used as control and the in vitro protein digestibility of the algae was expressed as a relative percentage to that of the sodium caseinate normalized at 100%.

3.5. Preparation of F. spiralis Protein Hydrolysate (FSPH)

The enzymatic reaction of the *F. spiralis* protein concentrate was carried out using two enzymes, cellulase followed by bromelain. One gram of protein concentrate sample was suspended and homogenized in 10 mL of ice-cold distilled water and each enzyme (substrate/enzyme ratio to 100:1, w/w) was individually added to the homogenate. For the enzymatic reaction was used cellulase at 50 °C and pH 4.5 (adjusted with 0.1 M HCl) followed by bromelain at 37 °C and pH 7.0 (adjusted with 0.5 M NaOH). The hydrolytic reaction was carried out for 20 h and after this period, the digestion solution was boiled for 10 min in order to inactivate the enzymes. The protein hydrolysate solution was centrifuged at 3000× *g* for 15 min, filtered through 0.45 μm filters, lyophilized in a freeze-drier and stored at −20 °C for further analysis.

3.6. Fractionation of FSPH by Ultrafiltration

The digested FSPH with cellulase and bromelain enzymes was further fractionated in a cell dialyzer system through three different ultrafiltration membranes with molecular weight cut-off (MWCO) of 1 and 3 kDa to obtain ultrafiltrates ($Fr_1 < 1$ kDa, 1 kDa $\leq Fr_2 < 3$ kDa and $Fr_3 \geq 3$ kDa). All the pooled FSPH fractions were lyophilized in a freeze-drier and assayed for ACE-inhibitory and antioxidant activities. The recovery yield of the ultrafiltration fractions was calculated using the gravimetric method.

3.7. Protein and Peptide Contents Analysis of FSPH Fractions

The protein content was determined by Bradford method [71] using BSA as the calibration standard and its peptide content was measured by OPA method [73] using glutathione as the calibration standard, according to Ghanbari et al. [46].

3.8. Amino Acids Composition of FSPH Fractions

The amino acids composition of FSPH fractions was determined according to Paiva et al. [3]. The dried FSPH fractions (0.5 mg) were placed in a small reaction vials, exposed to a stream of dry nitrogen, then capped and submitted to an acid hydrolysis at 100 °C for 24 h with 100 μL 6 N HCl containing 0.1% phenol for tyrosine protection. After cooling until room temperature, the samples were evaporated under a stream of dry nitrogen and then derivatized slowly by adding the mixture of acetyl chloride:isobutanol (1.25:5 mL, v/v, the reagent was obtained by adding the acetyl chloride to isobutanol precooled to −20 °C) and heating at 100 °C for 60 min. Next, the sample vials were opened and the mixtures exposed to a stream of dry nitrogen to remove excess reagent. After cooling in an ice bath, the samples were supplemented with 200 μL of acetonitrile and 50 μL of the derivatization reagent HFB-IBA, and heated again at 100 °C for 15 min. After evaporation of the excess reagent at 115 °C under a stream of dry nitrogen and cooling to room temperature, samples were dissolved in 300 μL of ethyl acetate and an aliquot (1 μL) was used for GC analysis. The GC analysis was performed using a Bruker GC model 450-GC gas chromatograph equipped with a split/splitless injector and a flame ionization detector (FID) using a wall-coated open tubular (WCOT) fused silica AT-Amino acid capillary column (25 m × 0.53 mm i.d., 1.2 μm film thickness) from Heliflex/Alltech (San Jose, CA, USA). The temperature started at 60 °C for 3 min, programmed at a rate of 4 °C/min to 210 °C and then held at this temperature for further 20 min. The injector and detector temperatures were held constants at 260 °C and 280 °C, respectively. Helium was the carrier gas at a flow rate of 28 cm/s.

3.9. Total Phenolic Content (TPC) Determination of FSPH Fractions

TPC was determined according to the method of Waterhouse [74] with slight modifications. An aliquot of 100 µL of FSPH fraction (2 mg/mL) was mixed with 1500 µL of distilled water and 100 µL of 2N FCR, homogenized in a vortex for 15 s and placed in dark for 3 min. Then, 300 µL of 10% Na_2CO_3 (w/v) was added to the mixture, homogenized and incubated for 5 min at 50 °C. The Abs values were measured at 760 nm. A blank sample was prepared by replacing the sample with Milli-Q water. The phloroglucinol (a basic structural unit of phlorotannins) was used as a standard and the results are expressed as mg of phloroglucinol equivalents (PE) per gram of dried FSPH fraction. A calibration curve was prepared using a concentration range of 50–300 µg/mL.

3.10. ACE-Inhibitory Activity Determination of FSPH Fractions

The determination of ACE-inhibitory activity was performed in vitro by RP-HPLC adapted from the spectrophotometric method described by Cushman and Cheung [75] with slight modifications [3]. This method is based on the liberation of hippuric acid from hippuryl-L-histidyl-L-leucine (Hip-His-Leu) catalyzed by ACE. For the assay, 42.5 µL of the sample solution (2 mg/mL) was pre-incubated at 37 °C for 5 min with 10 µL ACE (0.6 mU/mL) enzyme. The mixture was subsequently incubated at the same temperature for 60 min with 20 µL of the substrate (5 mM HHL in 10 µM zinc chloride containing 100 mM sodium trizma base and 300 mM NaCl at pH 8.3). The reaction was terminated by adding 12.5 µL of 5 M HCl. The percentage of ACE-inhibition was determined by an HPLC system from Waters equipped with a 626 pump and 600S controller coupled to a 486 tunable UV detector. An aliquot of 20 µL from the reaction mixture was analyzed on a reverse-phase Ultrasphere ODS analytical column (25 cm × 4.6 mm i.d., 5 µm particle size) (Beckman Coulter, Miami, FL, USA) using an isocratic elution of MeOH: ACN: 0.1% HCl (25:25:50, $v/v/v$) at a constant flow-rate of 0.6 mL/min and HA and HHL were detected by UV at 228 nm. The average value from three determinations at each concentration was used to calculate the ACE-inhibition (%) rate as follows: % ACE-inhibition = [B − A/B − C] × 100, where A is the absorbance (Abs) of HA generated in the presence of ACE-inhibitor, B the Abs of HA generated without ACE-inhibitor and C the Abs of HA generated without ACE (corresponding to HHL autolysis in the course of enzymatic assay). The IC_{50} value (mg/mL) was defined as the concentration of inhibitor required to reduce the HA peak by 50% (corresponding to 50% inhibition of ACE activity). The captopril was used as a positive control for ACE-inhibition.

3.11. Antioxidant Activity Assays on FSPH Fractions

3.11.1. DPPH Free Radical Scavenging Activity (FRSA) Assay

The FRSA of FSPH fractions was determined according to the method of Molyneux [76] with slight modifications. The FRSA of each FSPH fraction was tested by measuring their ability to quench DPPH. The DPPH, a stable free radical, is reduced changing the purple color of the DPPH radical solution to a bright yellow in the presence of antioxidants that possess hydrogen-donating or chain-breaking properties and the intensity of this can be monitored spectrophotometrically [77]. An aliquot of 250 µL of FSPH fraction with various concentrations (or BHT) was added to 250 µL of 100 mM DPPH solution. BHT was used as reference sample and a mixture without FSPH sample or BHT was used as the control. The Abs was measured at 517 nm after 30 min in the dark. The FRSA of FSPH fractions was calculated as a percentage of DPPH decoloration using the following equation: % FRSA = (1 − $Abs_{sample}/Abs_{control}$) × 100.

3.11.2. Ferrous Ion-Chelating (FIC) Activity Assay

Chelating ability of FSPH fractions was determined according to the modified method of Wang et al. [58], by measuring the inhibition of the Fe^{2+}–ferrozine complex formation. An aliquot of 100 µL of each FSPH fraction (concentration 2 mg/mL) was mixed with 135 µL of methanol plus 5 µL of 2 mM $FeCl_2$. The reaction was initiated by the addition of 10 µL of 5 mM ferrozine. After 10 min at room temperature, the Abs was determined at 562 nm. Methanol instead of ferrozine solution was used as a sample blank, which is used for error correction because of unequal color of the sample solutions. Methanol instead of sample solution was used as a control. Results are expressed as relative iron chelating activity compared with the unchelated (without ferrozine) Fe^{2+} reaction, and EDTA was used as reference standard. A lower Abs indicated a better FIC ability. The FIC ability was calculated as follows: % FIC ability = $[A_0 - (A_1 - A_2)]/A_0 \times 100$, where A_0 was the Abs of the control, A_1 was the Abs of the sample or standard and A_2 was the Abs of the blank.

3.11.3. Ferric Reducing Antioxidant Power (FRAP) Assay

The FRAP of FSPH fractions was determined according to the method of Oyaizu [78], and evaluated on the basis of their abilities to reduce Fe^{3+} complex to Fe^{2+}. An increased Abs value indicates an increased reducing power of the hydrolysate fractions. Each fraction (concentration range 12.5–100 µg/mL) in methanol (0.4 mL) was mixed with 0.4 mL of 300 mM of phosphate buffer (pH 6.6) plus 0.4 mL of potassium ferricyanide (1%, *w/v*) and the mixture was incubated at 50 °C for 20 min. After cooling down, 0.4 mL of TCA (10%, *w/v*) was added, and the mixture was centrifuged at $3000 \times g$ for 10 min. The upper layer (1 mL) was mixed with 1 mL of deionized water plus 0.2 mL of $FeCl_3$ (0.1% *w/v*), and the Abs was measured at 700 nm against a blank. The blank solution contained pure methanol instead of the methanolic FSPH fraction. BHT was used for comparison.

3.12. Statistical Analysis

All determinations were performed at least in triplicate and the results were expressed as means ± standard deviations (SD). The statistics analysis was performed using SPSS 17.0 (version 17, SPSS Inc., Chicago, IL, USA) and one-way analysis of variance test (ANOVA) was carried out to assess for any significant differences between the means. Differences between means at the 5% ($p < 0.05$) level were considered significant. Correlations between the parameters evaluated were obtained using Pearson's correlation coefficient (r).

4. Conclusions

Algae remain a relatively untapped source of compounds with ACE-inhibitory and antioxidant activities. To the best of our knowledge, this study revealed, for the first time, that enzymatic hydrolysate fractions with the aforementioned bifunctional properties could be efficiently generated from *F. spiralis* protein hydrolyzed by the cellulase–bromelain enzymes. The fraction with MW ≥3 kDa, obtained from this hydrolysate using ultrafiltration membranes, showed significantly higher recovery yield, ACE-inhibition and ferric reducing antioxidant power than the other fractions, and also showed strong scavenging of DPPH radical and ferrous ions (Fe^{2+}) chelating activity. The significant bioactivity of this fraction can be attributed to the high concentration of the potent active peptide sequences (even though the fraction contains peptides relatively large in size) and phenolic compounds (high-MW phlorotannins). Although additional research is needed on structural information of the bioactive compounds, overall results from this study indicate that the produced *F. spiralis* protein hydrolysate fractions can be promising natural sources to develop functional food ingredients for controlling hypertension and/or oxidative stress, the two major causes of cardiovascular diseases. However, in vivo studies are also needed to verify their physiological effects.

Acknowledgments: This study was financially supported by cE3c funding (Ref: UID/BIA/00329/2013). Lisete Paiva was supported by a doctoral grant (Ref: M3.1.2/F/014/2011) awarded by FRC (Fundo Regional da Ciência).

Author Contributions: Lisete Paiva designed the research project, performed the experimental work, analyzed the results and wrote the paper. Elisabete Lima, Ana Isabel Neto and José Baptista participated in the supervision process and critically revised the manuscript. All the authors approved the final manuscript.

Conflicts of Interest: The authors declare no conflict of interest.

References

1. Lordan, S.; Ross, R.P.; Stanton, C. Marine bioactives as functional food ingredients: Potential to reduce the incidence of chronic diseases. *Mar. Drugs* **2011**, *9*, 1056–1100. [PubMed]
2. Hata, Y.; Nakajima, K.; Uchida, J.I.; Hidaka, H.; Nakano, T. Clinical effects of brown seaweed, *Undaria pinnatifida* (*wakame*), on blood pressure in hypertensive subjects. *J. Clin. Biochem. Nutr.* **2001**, *30*, 43–53. [CrossRef]
3. Paiva, L.; Lima, E.; Neto, A.I.; Baptista, J. Isolation and characterization of angiotensin I-converting enzyme (ACE) inhibitory peptides from *Ulva rigida* C. Agardh protein hydrolysate. *J. Funct. Foods* **2016**, *26*, 65–76. [CrossRef]
4. Soffer, R.L. Angiotensin-converting enzyme and the regulation of vasoactive peptides. *Annu. Rev. Biochem.* **1976**, *45*, 73–94. [CrossRef] [PubMed]
5. Zhang, Y.; Lee, E.T.; Devereux, R.B.; Yeh, J.; Best, L.G.; Fabsitz, R.R.; Howard, B.V. Prehypertension, diabetes, and cardiovascular disease risk in a population-based sample: The strong heart study. *Hypertension* **2006**, *47*, 410–414. [CrossRef] [PubMed]
6. Andrews, P.R.; Carson, J.M.; Caselli, A.; Spark, M.J.; Woods, R. Conformational analysis and active site modelling of angiotensin-converting enzyme inhibitors. *J. Med. Chem.* **1985**, *28*, 393–399. [CrossRef] [PubMed]
7. Suetsuna, K. Purification and identification of angiotensin I-converting enzyme inhibitors from the red alga *Porphyra yezoensis*. *J. Mar. Biotechnol.* **1998**, *6*, 163–167. [PubMed]
8. Sato, M.; Hosokawa, T.; Yamaguchi, T.; Nakano, T.; Muramoto, K.; Kahara, T.; Funayama, K.; Kobayashi, A.; Nakano, T. Angiotensin I-converting enzyme inhibitory peptides derived from Wakame (*Undaria pinnatifida*) and their antihypertensive effect in spontaneously hypertensive rats. *J. Agric. Food Chem.* **2002**, *50*, 6245–6252. [CrossRef] [PubMed]
9. Paiva, L.; Lima, E.; Neto, A.I.; Baptista, J. Angiotensin I-converting enzyme (ACE) inhibitory activity of *Fucus spiralis* macroalgae and influence of the extracts storage temperature: A short report. *J. Pharm. Biomed. Anal.* **2016**, *131*, 503–507. [CrossRef] [PubMed]
10. Jung, H.A.; Hyun, S.K.; Kim, H.R.; Choi, J.S. Angiotensin-converting enzyme I inhibitory activity of phlorotannins from *Ecklonia stolonifera*. *Fish. Sci.* **2006**, *72*, 1292–1299. [CrossRef]
11. Wijesekara, I.; Kim, S.-K. Angiotensin-I-converting enzyme (ACE) inhibitors from marine resources: Prospects in the pharmaceutical industry. *Mar. Drugs* **2010**, *8*, 1080–1093. [CrossRef] [PubMed]
12. Wijesinghe, W.A.J.P.; Ko, S.-C.; Jeon, Y.-J. Effect of phlorotannins isolated from *Ecklonia cava* on angiotensin I-converting enzyme (ACE) inhibitory activity. *Nutr. Res. Pract.* **2011**, *5*, 93–100. [CrossRef] [PubMed]
13. Olivares-Molina, A.; Fernández, K. Comparison of different extraction techniques for obtaining extracts from brown seaweeds and their potential effects as angiotensin I-converting enzyme (ACE) inhibitors. *J. Appl. Phycol.* **2016**, *28*, 1295–1302. [CrossRef]
14. Catarino, M.D.; Silva, A.M.S.; Cardoso, S.M. Fucaceae: A source of bioactive phlorotannins. *Int. J. Mol. Sci.* **2017**, *18*, 1327. [CrossRef] [PubMed]
15. Harnedy, P.A.; FitzGerald, R.J. Bioactive proteins, peptides and amino acids from macroalgae. *J. Phycol.* **2011**, *47*, 218–232. [CrossRef] [PubMed]
16. Samarakoon, K.; Jeon, Y.-J. Bio-functionalities of proteins derived from marine algae—A review. *Food Res. Int.* **2012**, *48*, 948–960. [CrossRef]
17. Cian, R.E.; Alaiz, M.; Vioque, J.; Drago, S.R. Enzyme proteolysis enhanced extraction of ACE inhibitory and antioxidant compounds (peptides and polyphenols) from *Porphyra columbina* residual cake. *J. Appl. Phycol.* **2013**, *25*, 1197–1206. [CrossRef]

18. Oroian, M.; Escriche, I. Antioxidants: Characterization, natural sources, extraction and analysis. *Food Res. Int.* **2015**, *74*, 10–36. [CrossRef] [PubMed]

19. Korhonen, H.; Pihlanto, A. Food-derived bioactive peptides—Opportunities for designing future foods. *Curr. Pharm. Des.* **2003**, *9*, 1297–1308. [CrossRef] [PubMed]

20. Wijesinghe, W.A.; Jeon, Y.-J. Enzyme-assistant extraction (EAE) of bioactive components: A useful approach for recovery of industrially important metabolites from seaweeds: A review. *Fitoterapia* **2012**, *83*, 6–12. [CrossRef] [PubMed]

21. Neto, A.I.; Brotas, V.; Azevedo, J.M.N.; Patarra, R.F.; Álvaro, N.M.V.; Gameiro, C.; Prestes, A.C.L.; Nogueira, E.M. *Qualidade de Águas Costeiras do Grupo Oriental do Arquipélago dos Açores e Proposta de Monitorização*; Universidade dos Açores: Ponta Delgada, Portugal, 2009.

22. Neto, A.I.; Tittley, I.; Raposeiro, P.M. *Flora Marinha do Litoral dos Açores. Rocky Shore Marine Flora of the Azores*; Secretaria Regional do Ambiente e do Mar: Horta, Portugal, 2005.

23. Paiva, L.; Lima, E.; Patarra, R.F.; Neto, A.I.; Baptista, J. Edible Azorean macroalgae as source of rich nutrients with impact on human health. *Food Chem.* **2014**, *164*, 128–135. [CrossRef] [PubMed]

24. Cerantola, S.; Breton, F.; Ar Gall, E.; Deslandes, E. Co-occurrence and antioxidant activities of fucol and fucophlorethol classes of polymeric phenols in *Fucus spiralis*. *Bot. Mar.* **2006**, *49*, 347–351. [CrossRef]

25. Tierney, M.S.; Smyth, T.J.; Rai, D.K.; Soler-Vila, A.; Croft, A.K.; Brunton, N. Enrichment of polyphenol contents and antioxidant activities of Irish brown macroalgae using food-friendly techniques based on polarity and molecular size. *Food Chem.* **2013**, *139*, 753–761. [CrossRef] [PubMed]

26. Pinteus, S.; Silva, J.; Alves, C.; Horta, A.; Fino, N.; Inês Rodrigues, A.; Mendes, S.; Pedrosa, R. Cytoprotective effect of seaweeds with high antioxidant activity from the Peniche coast (Portugal). *Food Chem.* **2017**, *218*, 591–599. [CrossRef] [PubMed]

27. Fleurence, J. Seaweed proteins: Biochemical nutritional aspects and potential uses. *Trends Food Sci. Technol.* **1999**, *10*, 25–28. [CrossRef]

28. Quiroz-Castañeda, R.E.; Folch-Mallol, J.L. Hydrolysis of biomass mediated by cellulases for the production of sugars. In *Sustainable Degradation of Lignocellulosic Biomass-Techniques, Applications and Commercialization*; Chandel, A.K., da Silva, S.S., Eds.; InTech North America: New York, NY, USA, 2013.

29. Paiva, L.; Lima, E.; Neto, A.I.; Baptista, J. Screening for angiotensin I-converting enzyme (ACE) inhibitory activity of enzymatic hydrolysates obtained from Azorean macroalgae. *Arquipél. Life Mar. Sci.* **2015**, *32*, 11–17.

30. Elavarasan, K.; Kumar, V.N.; Shamasundar, B.A. Antioxidant and functional properties of fish protein hydrolysates from fresh water carp (*Catla catla*) as influenced by the nature of enzyme. *J. Food Process. Preserv.* **2014**, *38*, 1207–1214. [CrossRef]

31. Gajanan, P.G.; Elavarasan, K.; Shamasundar, B.A. Bioactive and functional properties of protein hydrolysates from fish frame processing waste using plant proteases. *Environ. Sci. Pollut. Res.* **2016**, *23*, 24901–24911. [CrossRef] [PubMed]

32. Auwal, S.M.; Zarei, M.; Abdul-Hamid, A.; Saari, N. Optimization of bromelain-aided production of angiotensin I-converting enzyme inhibitory hydrolysates from stone fish using response surface methodology. *Mar. Drugs* **2017**, *15*, 104. [CrossRef] [PubMed]

33. Chalé, F.G.H.; Ruiz, J.C.R.; Fernández, J.J.A.; Ancona, D.A.B.; Campos, M.R.S. ACE inhibitory, hypotensive and antioxidant peptide fractions from *Mucuna pruriens* proteins. *Process Biochem.* **2014**, *49*, 1691–1698. [CrossRef]

34. Udenigwe, C.C.; Aluko, R.E. Chemometric analysis of the amino acid requirements of antioxidant food protein hydrolysates. *Int. J. Mol. Sci.* **2011**, *12*, 3148–3161. [CrossRef] [PubMed]

35. Fleurence, J. Seaweed proteins. In *Proteins in Food Processing*; Yada, R.Y., Ed.; Woodhead Publishing Limited: Cambridge, UK, 2004; pp. 197–213.

36. Ge, Y.; Sun, A.; Ni, Y.; Cai, T. Study and development of a defatted wheat germ nutritive noodle. *Eur. Food Res. Technol.* **2001**, *212*, 344–348. [CrossRef]

37. Athukorala, Y.; Jeon, Y.J. Screening for angiotensin I-converting enzyme inhibitory activity of *Ecklonia cava*. *J. Food Sci. Nutr.* **2005**, *10*, 134–139. [CrossRef]

38. Tierney, M.S.; Soler-vila, A.; Croft, A.K.; Hayes, M. Antioxidant activity of the brown macroalgae *Fucus spiralis* Linnaeus harvested from the west coast of Ireland. *Curr. Res. J. Biol. Sci.* **2013**, *5*, 81–90.

39. Wang, T.; Jónsdóttir, R.; Liu, H.; Gu, L.; Kristinsson, H.G.; Raghavan, S.; Ólafsdóttir, G. Antioxidant capacities of phlorotannins extracted from the brown algae *Fucus vesiculosus*. *J. Agric. Food Chem.* **2012**, *60*, 5874–5883. [CrossRef] [PubMed]

40. Steevensz, A.J.; MacKinnon, S.L.; Hankinson, R.; Craft, C.; Connan, S.; Stengel, D.B.; Melanson, J.E. Profiling phlorotannins in brown macroalgae by liquid chromatography-high resolution mass spectrometry. *Phytochem. Anal.* **2012**, *23*, 547–553. [CrossRef] [PubMed]

41. Ferreres, F.; Lopes, G.; Gil-Izquierdo, A.; Andrade, P.B.; Sousa, C.; Mouga, T.; Valentão, P. Phlorotannin extracts from Fucales characterized by HPLC-DAD-ESI-MS^n: Approaches to hyaluronidase inhibitory capacity and antioxidant properties. *Mar. Drugs* **2012**, *10*, 2766–2781. [CrossRef] [PubMed]

42. Zhao, Y.; Li, B.; Dong, S.; Liu, Z.; Zhao, X.; Wang, J.; Zeng, M. A novel ACE inhibitory peptide isolated from *Acaudina molpadioidea* hydrolysate. *Peptides* **2009**, *30*, 1028–1033. [CrossRef] [PubMed]

43. Hong, L.G.; Wei, L.G.; Liu, H.; Hui, S.Y. Mung-bean protein hydrolysates obtained with Alcalase exhibit angiotensin I-converting enzyme inhibitory activity. *Food Sci. Technol. Int.* **2005**, *11*, 281–287.

44. Wilson, J.; Hayes, M.; Carney, B. Angiotensin-I-converting enzyme and prolyl endopeptidase inhibitory peptides from natural sources with a focus on marine processing by-products. *Food Chem.* **2011**, *129*, 235–244. [CrossRef]

45. Segura-Campos, M.R.; Peralta-González, F.; Castellanos-Ruelas, A.; Chel-Guerrero, L.A.; Betancur-Ancona, D.A. Effect of *Jatropha curcas* peptide fractions on the angiotensin I-converting enzyme inhibitory activity. *Biomed. Res. Int.* **2013**. [CrossRef] [PubMed]

46. Ghanbari, R.; Zarei, M.; Ebrahimpour, A.; Abdul-Hamid, A.; Ismail, A.; Saari, N. Angiotensin-I converting enzyme (ACE) inhibitory and anti-oxidant activities of sea cucumber (*Actinopyga lecanora*) hydrolysates. *Int. J. Mol. Sci.* **2015**, *16*, 28870–28885. [CrossRef] [PubMed]

47. Liu, J.-C.; Hsu, F.-L.; Tsai, J.-C.; Chan, P.; Liu, J.Y.; Thomas, G.N.; Tomlinson, B.; Lo, M.-Y.; Lin, J.-Y. Antihypertensive effects of tannins isolated from traditional Chinese herbs as non-specific inhibitors of angiotensin converting enzyme. *Life Sci.* **2003**, *73*, 1543–1555. [CrossRef]

48. Wang, T.; Jónsdóttir, R.; Kristinsson, H.G.; Hreggvidsson, G.O.; Jónsson, J.O.; Thorkelsson, G.; Ólafsdóttir, G. Enzyme-enhanced extraction of antioxidant ingredients from red algae *Palmaria palmata*. *LWT—Food Sci. Technol.* **2010**, *43*, 1387–1393. [CrossRef]

49. Fan, J.; He, J.; Zhuang, Y.; Sun, L. Purification and identification of antioxidant peptides from enzymatic hydrolysates of Tilapia (*Oreochromis niloticus*) frame protein. *Molecules* **2012**, *17*, 12836–12850. [CrossRef] [PubMed]

50. Udenigwe, C.C.; Lu, Y.-L.; Han, C.-H.; Hou, W.-C.; Aluko, R.E. Flaxseed protein-derived peptide fractions: Antioxidant properties and inhibition of lipopolysaccharide-induced nitric oxide production in murine macrophages. *Food Chem.* **2009**, *116*, 277–284. [CrossRef]

51. Chen, H.-M.; Muramoto, K.; Yamauchi, F.; Fujimoto, K.; Nokihara, K. Antioxidative properties of histidine-containing peptides designed from peptide fragments found in the digests of a soybean protein. *J. Agric. Food. Chem.* **1998**, *46*, 49–53. [CrossRef] [PubMed]

52. Guo, H.; Kouzuma, Y.; Yonekura, M. Structures and properties of antioxidative peptides derived from royal jelly protein. *Food Chem.* **2009**, *113*, 238–245. [CrossRef]

53. Rajapakse, N.; Mendis, E.; Jung, W.-K.; Je, J.-Y.; Kim, S.-K. Purification of a radical scavenging peptide from fermented mussel sauce and its antioxidant properties. *Food. Res. Int.* **2005**, *38*, 175–182. [CrossRef]

54. Nimalaratne, C.; Bandara, N.; Wu, J. Purification and characterization of antioxidant peptides from enzymatically hydrolyzed chicken egg white. *Food Chem.* **2015**, *188*, 467–472. [CrossRef] [PubMed]

55. Alemán, A.; Pérez-Santín, E.; Bordenave-Juchereau, S.; Arnaudin, I.; Gómez-Guillén, M.C.; Montero, P. Squid gelatin hydrolysates with antihypertensive, anticancer and antioxidant activity. *Food Res. Int.* **2011**, *44*, 1044–1051. [CrossRef]

56. Heffernan, N.; Smyth, T.J.; Soler-Villa, A.; Fitzgerald, R.J.; Brunton, N.P. Phenolic content and antioxidant activity of fractions obtained from selected Irish macroalgae species (*Laminaria digitata, Fucus serratus, Gracilaria gracilis* and *Codium fragile*). *J. Appl. Phycol.* **2015**, *27*, 519–530. [CrossRef]

57. Kim, K.N.; Heo, S.-J.; Song, C.B.; Lee, J.; Heo, M.S.; Yeo, I.K.; Kang, K.; Hyun, J.W.; Jeon, Y.-J. Protective effect of *Ecklonia cava* enzymatic extracts on hydrogen peroxide-induced cell damage. *Process Biochem.* **2006**, *41*, 2393–2401. [CrossRef]

58. Wang, T.; Jónsdóttir, R.; Ólafsdóttir, G. Total phenolic compounds, radical scavenging and metal chelation of extracts from Icelandic seaweeds. *Food Chem.* **2009**, *116*, 240–248. [CrossRef]

59. Torres-Fuentes, C.; Alaiz, M.; Vioque, J. Affinity purification and characterisation of chelating peptides from chickpea protein hydrolysates. *Food Chem.* **2011**, *129*, 485–490. [CrossRef]

60. Girgih, A.T.; Udenigwe, C.C.; Aluko, R.E. In vitro antioxidant properties of hemp seed (*Cannabis sativa* L.) protein hydrolysate fractions. *J. Am. Oil Chem. Soc.* **2011**, *88*, 381–389. [CrossRef]

61. Senevirathne, M.; Kim, S.-H.; Siriwardhana, N.; Ha, J.-H.; Lee, K.-W.; Jeon, Y.-J. Antioxidant potential of *Ecklonia cava* on reactive oxygen species scavenging, metal chelating, reducing power and lipid peroxidation inhibition. *Rev. Agaroquim. Tecnol. Aliment.* **2006**, *12*, 27–38.

62. Santoso, J.; Yoshie-Stark, Y.; Suzuki, T. Anti-oxidant activity of methanol extracts from Indonesian seaweeds in an oil emulsion model. *Fish. Sci.* **2004**, *70*, 183–188. [CrossRef]

63. Duh, P.-D. Antioxidant activity of burdock (*Arctium lappa* Linné): It's scavenging effect on free radical and active oxygen. *J. Am. Oil Chem. Soc.* **1998**, *75*, 455–461. [CrossRef]

64. Chandini, S.-K.; Ganesan, P.; Bhaskar, N. In vitro antioxidant activities of three selected brown seaweeds of India. *Food Chem.* **2008**, *107*, 707–713. [CrossRef]

65. Ganesan, P.; Kumar, C.S.; Bhaskar, N. Antioxidant properties of methanol extract and its solvent fractions obtained from selected Indian red seaweeds. *Bioresour. Technol.* **2008**, *99*, 2717–2723. [CrossRef] [PubMed]

66. Zubia, M.; Fabre, M.S.; Kerjean, V.; Lann, K.L.; Stiger-Pouvreau, V.; Fauchon, M.; Deslandes, E. Antioxidant and antitumoural activities of some Phaeophyta from Brittany coasts. *Food Chem.* **2009**, *116*, 693–701. [CrossRef]

67. Vinayak, R.C.; Sabu, A.S.; Chatterji, A. Bio-prospecting of a few brown seaweeds for their cytotoxic and antioxidant activities. *Evid. Based Complement. Altern. Med.* **2011**. [CrossRef] [PubMed]

68. Babbar, N.; Oberoi, H.S.; Uppal, D.S.; Patil, R.T. Total phenolic content and antioxidant capacity of extracts obtained from six important fruit residues. *Food Res. Int.* **2011**, *44*, 391–396. [CrossRef]

69. Pal, R.; Rai, J.P. Phytochelatins: Peptides involved in heavy metal detoxification. *Appl. Biochem. Biotechnol.* **2010**, *160*, 945–963. [CrossRef] [PubMed]

70. Wong, K.H.; Cheung, P.C.K.; Ang, P.O., Jr. Nutritional evaluation of protein concentrates isolated from two red seaweeds: *Hypnea charoides* and *Hypnea japonica* in growing rats. *Hydrobiologia* **2004**, *512*, 271–278. [CrossRef]

71. Bradford, M.M. A rapid and sensitive method for the quantitation of microgram quantities of protein utilizing the principle of protein-dye binding. *Anal. Biochem.* **1976**, *72*, 248–254. [CrossRef]

72. Paiva, L.; Lima, E.; Neto, A.I.; Massimo, M.; Baptista, J. Nutritional and functional bioactivity value of selected Azorean macroalgae: *Ulva compressa*, *Ulva rigida*, *Gelidium microdon*, and *Pterocladiella capillacea*. *J. Food Sci.* **2017**, *82*, 1757–1764. [CrossRef] [PubMed]

73. Church, F.C.; Swaisgood, H.E.; Porter, D.H.; Catignani, G.L. Spectrophotometric assay using *O*-phthaldialdehyde for determination of proteolysis in milk and isolated milk proteins. *J. Dairy Sci.* **1983**, *66*, 1219–1227. [CrossRef]

74. Waterhouse, A.L. Determination of total phenolics. In *Current Protocols in Food Analytical Chemistry*; Wrolstad, R.E., Ed.; John Wiley & Sons: New York, NY, USA, 2002.

75. Cushman, D.W.; Cheung, H.S. Spectrophotometric assay and properties of the angiotensin-converting enzyme of rabbit lung. *Biochem. Pharmacol.* **1971**, *20*, 1637–1648. [CrossRef]

76. Molyneux, P. The use of the stable free radical diphenylpicrylhydrazyl (DPPH) for estimating antioxidant activity. *Songklanakarin J. Sci. Technol.* **2004**, *26*, 211–219.

77. Corrêa, A.P.; Daroit, D.J.; Coelho, J.; Meira, S.M.; Lopes, F.C.; Risso, P.H.; Brandelli, A. Antioxidant, antihypertensive and antimicrobial properties of ovine milk caseinate hydrolyzed with a microbial protease. *J. Sci. Food Agric.* **2011**, *91*, 2247–2254. [CrossRef] [PubMed]

78. Oyaizu, M. Studies on products of browning reactions: Antioxidative activities of products of browning reaction prepared from glucosamine. *Jpn. J. Nutr.* **1986**, *44*, 307–315. [CrossRef]

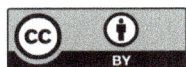

Review

Terpenoids from Octocorals of the Genus *Pachyclavularia*

Yu-Chia Chang [1,2,3,4], Jyh-Horng Sheu [4,*], Yang-Chang Wu [5,6,7,*] and Ping-Jyun Sung [1,4,5,8,9,*]

[1] National Museum of Marine Biology and Aquarium, Pingtung 944, Taiwan; jay0404@gmail.com
[2] Greenhouse Systems Technology Center, Central Region Campus, Industrial Technology Research Institute, Nantou 540, Taiwan
[3] Forcean Marine International Corporation, Kaohsiung 800, Taiwan
[4] Department of Marine Biotechnology and Resources, National Sun Yat-sen University, Kaohsiung 804, Taiwan
[5] Graduate Institute of Natural Products, Kaohsiung Medical University, Kaohsiung 807, Taiwan
[6] Research Center for Natural Products and Drug Development, Kaohsiung Medical University, Kaohsiung 807, Taiwan
[7] Department of Medical Research, Kaohsiung Medical University Hospital, Kaohsiung 807, Taiwan
[8] Graduate Institute of Marine Biology, National Dong Hwa University, Pingtung 944, Taiwan
[9] Chinese Medicine Research and Development Center, China Medical University Hospital, Taichung 404, Taiwan
* Correspondence: sheu@mail.nsysu.edu.tw (J.-H.S.); yachwu@kmu.edu.tw (Y.-C.W.); pjsung@nmmba.gov.tw (P.-J.S.); Tel.: +886-7-525-2000 (ext. 5030) (J.-H.S.); +886-7-312-1101 (ext. 5347) (Y.-C.W.); +886-8-882-5037 (P.-J.S.); Fax: +886-7-525-5020 (J.-H.S.); +886-7-311-4773 (Y.-C.W.); +886-8-882-5087 (P.-J.S.)

Received: 2 November 2017; Accepted: 4 December 2017; Published: 5 December 2017

Abstract: In this paper, we reviewed natural compounds isolated from octocorals belonging to the genus *Pachyclavularia*, including 20 cembrane-, 39 briarane-, and eight briarellin-related diterpenoids, and one secosterol. The chemical constituents of these 68 secondary metabolites, and their names, structures, and bioactivities, along with studies of their biological activities, are summarized in this review. Based on the literature, many of these compounds possess bioactivities, including anti-inflammation properties, cytotoxicity, and ichthyotoxicity, suggesting that they may have the potential to be developed into biomedical agents for treatment.

Keywords: *Pachyclavularia*; octocoral; cembrane; briarane; briarellin; secosterol; bioactivity

1. Introduction

Octocorals of the genus *Pachyclavularia* (phylum Cnidaria, class Anthozoa, order Alcyonacea, family Briareidae) [1], which originally belonged to the family Tubiporidae [2], distributed in the subtropical and tropical waters of the Indo-Pacific Ocean, have been investigated. Since the initial study in 1979 discovered a cembranoid diterpene, pachyclavulariadiol (**1**), from the Australian octocoral *P. violacea* [3], subsequent studies over the past few decades have yielded a series of interesting secondary metabolites, particularly diterpenoids originally synthesized from cyclized cembranoids, including briarane- and briarellin-related analogues (Scheme 1) [4]. In this article, we have listed the different types of compounds isolated from two Indo-Pacific octocorals, *Pachyclavularia violacea* (Scheme 1) and *Pachyclavularia* sp., and summarized their chemical constituents and research into the biological activities of these metabolites.

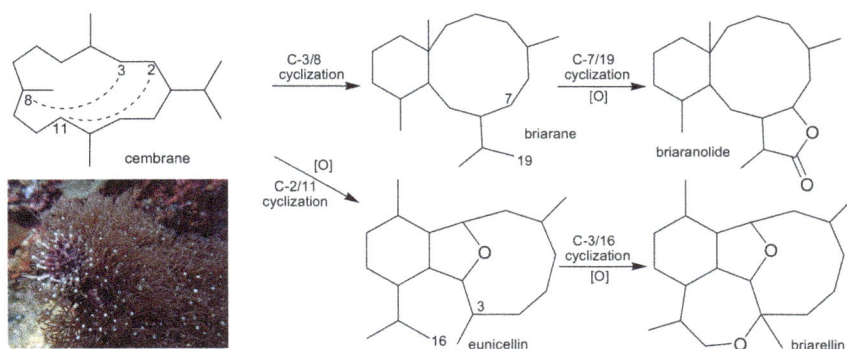

Scheme 1. Octocoral *P. violacea* and the proposed biosynthetic pathways of the cembrane, briarane, and briarellin carbon skeletons [4].

2. Cembranoids from *Pachyclavularia violacea* (Quoy and Gaimard, 1833) (=*Clavularia violacea, Briareum violaceum*)

The *Pachyclavularia* genus includes one very common species, *Pachyclavularia violacea* [2,3]. Bowden and colleagues [3] isolated several compounds, including three new cembrane-type diterpenes, pachyclavulariadiol (**1**), and its naturally-derived mono- and di-acetylated derivatives (**2** and **3**), from octocoral *P. violacea* collected in Australia (Figure 1). The study also established the structures, including the relative configurations, of new furanocembranoids **1**–**3** and determined the configuration of **1** by spectroscopic/chemical methods and X-ray diffraction, respectively.

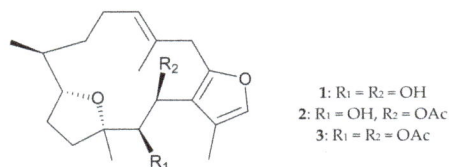

1: $R_1 = R_2 = OH$
2: $R_1 = OH, R_2 = OAc$
3: $R_1 = R_2 = OAc$

Figure 1. Structures of pachyclavulariadiol (**1**) and its natural mono- and di-acetylated derivatives **2** and **3**.

In 1989, Inman and Crews [5] reported the isolation of a new cembranolide from *P. violacea* collected from Vanuatu waters, and named the compound pachyclavularolide (**4**) (Figure 2). Later, the structure of **4**, including the relative configuration, was determined using spectroscopic methods and molecular mechanics calculations, and further confirmed by single-crystal X-ray analyses in a study by Sheu et al. [6]. The former study was the first to present a detailed conformational analysis of a 14-membered cembrane ring [5].

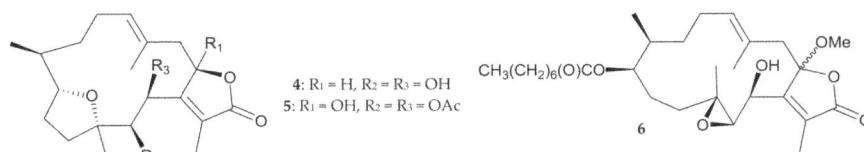

4: $R_1 = H, R_2 = R_3 = OH$
5: $R_1 = OH, R_2 = R_3 = OAc$

$CH_3(CH_2)_6(O)CO$

Figure 2. Structures of pachyclavularolide (**4**) and pachyclavulariolides E (**5**) and F (**6**).

Two new cembranes, pachyclavulariolides E (**5**) and F (**6**) (Figure 2), were isolated from *P. violacea* samples collected from waters off Madang in Papua New Guinea in 2000 [7]. The structures of **5** and **6**, including the relative configurations, which were elucidated from spectroscopic data [7], and the structure, including the relative configuration of **5**, was further confirmed from single-crystal X-ray analysis by Sheu et al. [6]. A cytotoxic assay showed that compound **6** had an IC$_{50}$ value of 1.0 µg/mL in the treatment of murine leukemia P388 cells [7], though this compound was claimed to be an artifact due to methanol used in the extraction procedure [7].

Twelve new cembranolides, pachyclavulariolides G–R (**7–18**) (Figure 3), and two known analogues, pachyclavulariolide (**4**) and pachyclavulariolide E (**5**) [5,7] (Figure 2), were obtained from *P. violacea* specimens collected from Kenting Coast, Taiwan [6,8]. The structures, including the relative configurations, of cembranolides **7–18** were established by spectroscopic/chemical methods [6,8], and the structures of **4**, **5**, **7**, and **8** were also verified by single-crystal analyses [6]. However, the hydroxy group at C-2 in briarane **11** was still unconfirmed at that stage [6], and information regarding the reasonable biosynthetic pathway suggested that briarane **12** could be the precursor of briarane **16** [8]. Cytotoxic assays revealed that pachyclavulariolide K (**11**) had ED$_{50}$ values of 2.8, 3.3, 6.7, and 7.6 µg/mL against P388 (mouse lymphoma), HT-29 (human colorectal adenocarcinoma), A549 (human epithelial carcinoma), and KB cells (human nasopharynx carcinoma), respectvively, while pachyclavulariolides E (**5**), I (**9**), J (**10**), and M (**13**) had ED$_{50}$ values against P388 cells of 4.0, 1.3, 2.5, and 3.2 µg/mL, respectively [6,8].

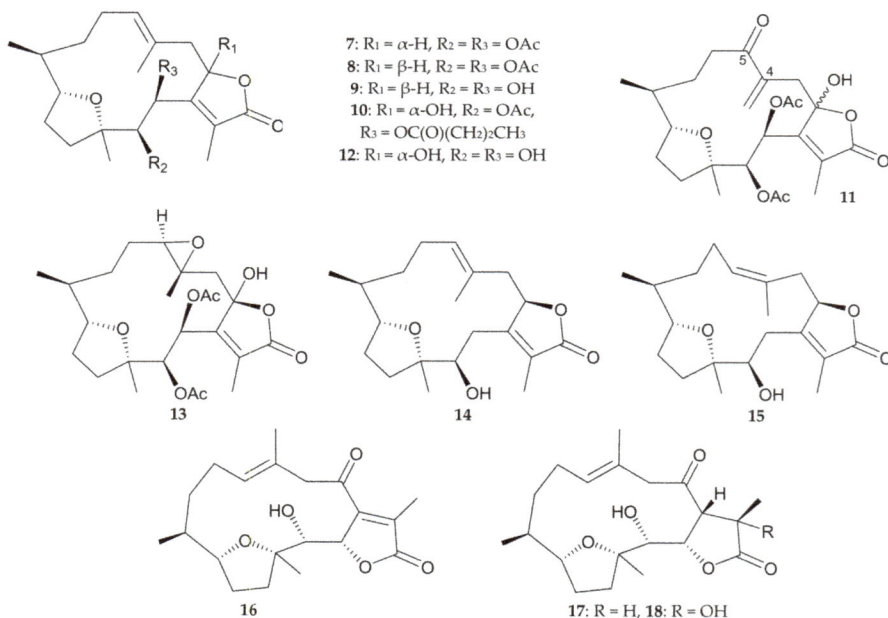

7: R$_1$ = α-H, R$_2$ = R$_3$ = OAc
8: R$_1$ = β-H, R$_2$ = R$_3$ = OAc
9: R$_1$ = β-H, R$_2$ = R$_3$ = OH
10: R$_1$ = α-OH, R$_2$ = OAc,
R$_3$ = OC(O)(CH$_2$)$_2$CH$_3$
12: R$_1$ = α-OH, R$_2$ = R$_3$ = OH

17: R = H, 18: R = OH

Figure 3. Structures of pachyclavulariolides G–R (**7–18**).

A new cytotoxic cembranoid, claviolide (**19**) (Figure 4), was isolated from the dichloromethane extract of *Clavularia violacea*, collected at a depth of 5–6 m off Green Island, Taiwan. The structure, including the relative configuration, of **19** was established using a spectroscopic approach, and this compound was found to exhibit significant cytotoxicity towards P388 and HT-29 tumor cells, with ED$_{50}$ values of 0.84 and 0.38 µg/mL, respectively [9].

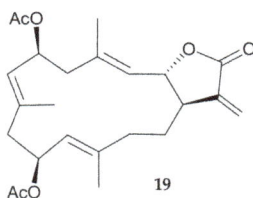

Figure 4. Structure of claviolide (**19**).

Chang and coworkers isolated a new cembranoid, briaviodiol A (**20**) (Figure 5), from the organic extract of *Briareum violaceum* [2] collected off Pingtung Coast, Southern Taiwan, and confirmed its structure, including the relative configuration, by single-crystal X-ray diffraction analysis [10].

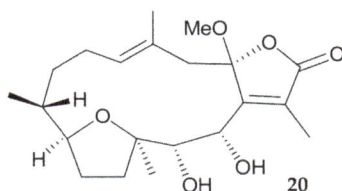

Figure 5. Structure of briaviodiol A (**20**).

Interestingly, with the exception of cembranoids **6** (pachyclavulariolide F) and **19** (claviolide), cembranoids (18/20) from *P. violacea* have been found to possess a tetrahydrofuran moiety, and these furanocembranoids are likely to be chemical markers of cembranoids obtained from *P. violacea*. Among the furanocembranoids, the α,β-unsaturated ketone moiety in pachyclavulariolide K (**11**) seems to enhance cytotoxicity toward various tumor cells.

3. Briaranes from *Pachyclavularia* sp. and *Pachyclavularia violacea*

Uchio and colleagues [11] identified three new unnamed briaranes, **21–23** (Figure 6), from specimens of the octocoral *Pachyclavularia* sp. collected off the Great Barrier Reef, Australia. The authors established the structures of **21–23**, including the relative configurations, using a spectroscopic approach, and also found that briarane **21** exhibited ichthyotoxicity towards the mosquito fish *Gambusia affinis*.

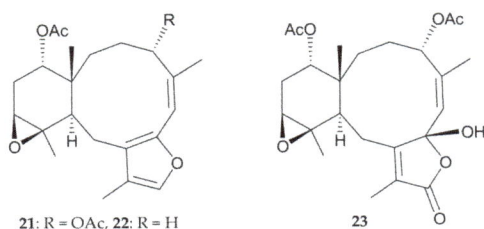

21: R = OAc, **22**: R = H   **23**

Figure 6. Structures of briaranes **21–23**.

Five briarane diterpenoids, including three new metabolites 2β-acetoxy-2-(debutyryloxy)-stecholide E (**24**), 9-deacetylstylatulide lactone (**25**), and 4β-acetoxy-9-deacetylstylatulide lactone (**26**), along with two known metabolites, brianthein W (**27**) [12] and 9-deacetylbriareolide H (**28**) [13,14]

(Figure 7), were isolated from a Taiwanese soft coral *Briareum* sp., which was originally identified as *Pachyclavularia violacea* collected off the coast of Kenting, Taiwan [15]. The structures of new briaranes **24–26**, including the relative configurations, were established by chemical/spectroscopic methods. Cytotoxic assays were performed on briaranes **24–28** to assess their toxicity against P388, HT-29, KB, and A549 tumor cells, and the results showed that all briaranes except **26** exhibited cytotoxicity against P388 cells, with ED_{50} values of 0.61, 1.12, 0.76 and 0.28 µg/mL, respectively [15], indicating that the acetoxy group at C-4 in **26** redeuce the cytotoxicity. Briaranes **25** and **28** showed cytotoxicity towards HT-29 and KB cells, with ED_{50} values of 1.79 and 0.27 µg/mL, respectively [15]. The cytotoxicities of 9-hydroxybriaranes **24**, **25**, and **28** were not significantly different to their corresponding 9-acetyl derivatives, 2β-acetoxy-2-(debutyryloxy)-stecholide E acetate, stylatulide lactone [16], and briareolide H [13], respectively [15].

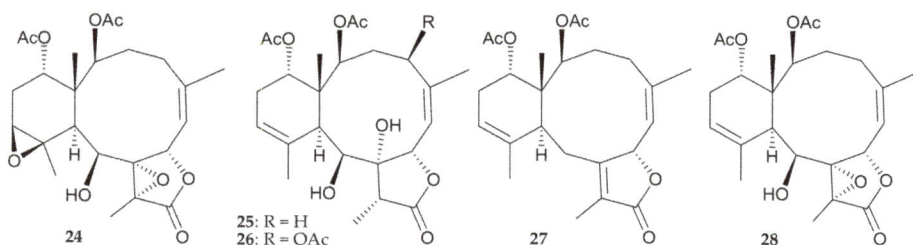

Figure 7. Structures of 2β-acetoxy-2-(debutyryloxy)stecholide E (**24**), 9-deacetylstylatulide lactone (**25**), 4β-acetoxy-9-deacetylstylatulide lactone (**26**), brianthein W (**27**), and 9-deacetylbriareolide H (**28**).

In 2000, Xu et al. [7] isolated four new briarane derivatives, pachyclavulariolides A–D (**29–32**) (Figure 8), from *P. violacea* specimens collected from reefs off Madang, Papua New Guinea. The authors used a spectroscopic approach to determine the structures, including the relative configurations, of **29–32**, and further employed single-crystal X-ray diffraction analysis to identify the structure, including the relative configuration, of briarane **30** (pachyclavulariolide B). They also found that briaranes **29–32** were the first briaranes of this type to possess an 11,14-ether bridge that resulted in an oxanorbornane structure.

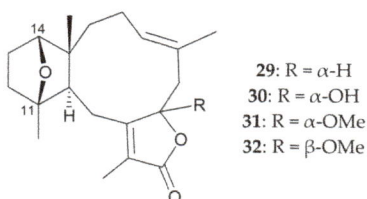

29: R = α-H
30: R = α-OH
31: R = α-OMe
32: R = β-OMe

Figure 8. Structures of pachyclavulariolides A–D (**29–32**).

Research by a group in Japan identified nine new briaranes, pachyclavulides A–I (**33–41**) (Figure 9), from *P. violacea* collected off Okinawa, and determined their structures, including the relative configurations, using spectroscopic methods [17,18]. The absolute configuration of pachyclavulide A (**33**) was determined by single-crystal X-ray diffraction analysis of its *p*-bromobenzoyl ester [17]. Pachyclavulides B (**34**) and E (**37**) were found to show cytotoxicity against human central neural system (CNS) SNB-75 and A549 (human alveolar epithelial carcinoma) tumor cells, with GI_{50} values of 5.2 and 5.1 µM, respectively [18] and pachyclavulide C (**35**) was not cytotoxic toward SNB-75 cells. It seems that the hydroxy group at C-16 in briarane **34** will enhance the cytotoxicity. Enantioselective preparation of the six-membered ring of pachyclavulide B (**34**) was also achieved [19].

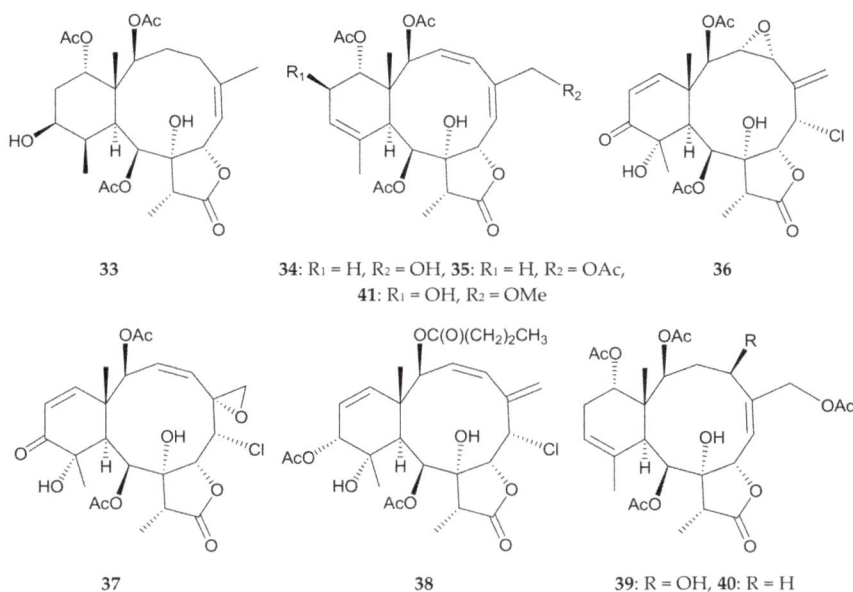

Figure 9. Structures of pachyclavulides A–I (**33–41**).

In addition, another group of researchers isolated four new briaranes, brianodins A–D (**42–45**), from soft coral identified as *Pachyclavularia* sp. from Okinawa, Japan [20]. They established the structures, including the relative configurations, of briaranes **42–45** by interpretation of spectroscopic data, and determined the absolute configurations of brianodins C (**44**) and D (**45**) by the modified Mosher's method (Figure 10). The 1,2-diol moiety at C-8 and C-17 in **43–45** is rarely found in briarane analogues [21–26].

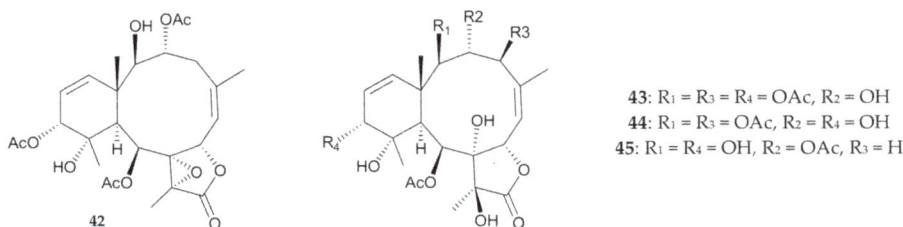

Figure 10. Structures of brianodins A–D (**42–45**).

Sixteen briarane analogues, including ten new metabolites briaviolides A–J (**46–55**), along with six known briaranes, solenolides A (**56**) and D (**57**) [27], excavatolide A (**58**) [28], briaexcavatolide I (**59**) [29] (Figure 11), 4β-acetoxy-9-deacetylstulatulide lactone (**26**) and 9-deacetylstylatulide lactone (**25**) [15] (Figure 7), were isolated from *Briareum violaceum* [2] collected in the waters of Taiwan [30]. Using spectroscopic/chemical methods, the structures, including the relative configurations, of new briaranes **46–55** were determined, and the absolute configuration of briaviolide A (**46**) was further confirmed by X-ray crystallographic analysis [30]. In anti-inflammatory activity assays, briaviolides E (**50**) and I (**54**) were found to possess inhibitory effects against the production of superoxide anions by human neutrophils in vitro (inhibition rates = 34.17% and 28.66%, respectively), and inhibited the release of elastase (inhibition rates = 26.03% and 28.81%, respectively) at a concentration of 10 µg/mL; while the monobenzoyl derivative of 46 was found to possess selective activity to inhibit elastase release (inhibition rate = 28.60%) at a concentration of 10 µg/mL [30]. By comparison of the structure-activity relationships between briaranes 53 (briaviolide H) and 54 (briaviolide I), indicating that the hydroperoxy group at C-12 in 54 enhance the activity to inhibit the elastase release and the generation of superoxide anions.

A study performed by Cheng et al. revised the structure of solenolide D (57) [31], and this compound was later found to be a potent anti-inflammatory agent with an efficacy comparable to that of indomethacin [27]. Potency in excess of a 70% reduction of edema was observed at a concentration of approximately 15 µg/per ear (mouse ear assay) [27].

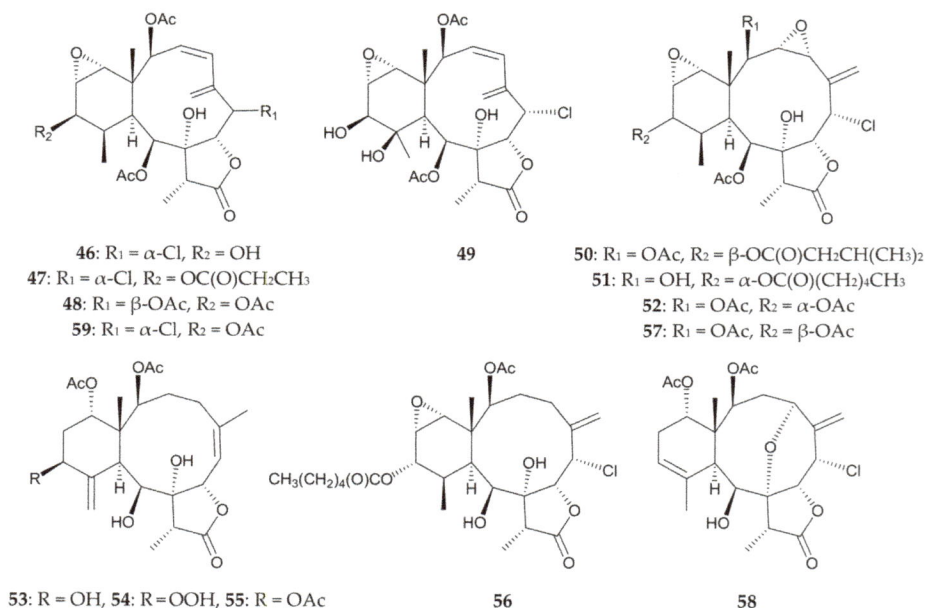

46: R₁ = α-Cl, R₂ = OH
47: R₁ = α-Cl, R₂ = OC(O)CH₂CH₃
48: R₁ = β-OAc, R₂ = OAc
59: R₁ = α-Cl, R₂ = OAc

49

50: R₁ = OAc, R₂ = β-OC(O)CH₂CH(CH₃)₂
51: R₁ = OH, R₂ = α-OC(O)(CH₂)₄CH₃
52: R₁ = OAc, R₂ = α-OAc
57: R₁ = OAc, R₂ = β-OAc

53: R = OH, 54: R = OOH, 55: R = OAc

56

58

Figure 11. Structures of briaviolides A–J (46–55), solenolides A (56) and D (57), excavatolide A (58), and briaexcavatolide I (59).

4. Briarellins from *Pachyclavularia violacea*

Eight novel briarellins, including pachyclavulariaenones A–G (60–66) [32,33] and secopachy-clavulariaenone A (67) [6] (Figure 12), were isolated from *P. violacea* collected off Kenting Coast, Taiwan. Pachyclavulariaenone B (61) was also isolated from *P. violacea* specimens collected in the Togian Islands near Sulawesi Island, Indonesia [34]. The structures, including the relative configurations, of briarellins 60–67 were established by spectroscopic methods, and the structures, including the relative configurations, of briarellins 62 (pachyclavulariaenone C) [32] and 65 (pachyclavulariaenone F) [33] were further confirmed by single-crystal X-ray diffraction analyses. Briarellins 60–67 were found to be unprecedented examples of this type of compound, as they possess a six-membered carbocyclic ring *cis*-fused to both the ten-membered carbocyclic ring and seven-membered ether ring, making three ring-junction protons *cis* to each other [6,32,33]. Cytotoxic assays revealed that pachyclavulariaenone G (66) exhibited cytotoxicity towards P388 and HT-29 tumor cells, with ED₅₀ values of 0.2 and 3.2 µg/mL, respectively [33]. It is obvious to note that the hydroxy groups at C-4 and C-6 in 66 caused this compound to be more cytotoxic than its analogues 62, 64, and 65.

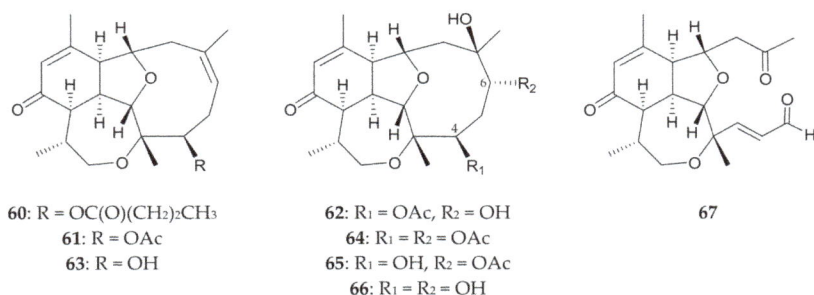

Figure 12. Structures of pachyclavulariaenones A–G (**60–66**) and secopachyclavulariaenone A (**67**).

5. Secosterol from *Pachyclavularia violacea*

A new 9,11-secosterol, (24*S**)-3β,11-dihydroxy-5β,6β-epoxy-24-methyl-9,11-secocholestan-9-one (**68**) (Figure 13), was isolated from *P. violacea* specimens collected off the Togian Islands, Indonesia, and its structure, including the relative configurations, was elucidated on the basis of spectroscopic data [34].

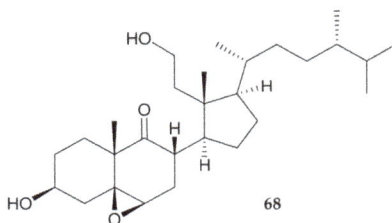

Figure 13. Structure of secosterol **68**.

6. Conclusions

Ever since pachyclavulariadiol (**1**) was obtained from a specimen of the octocoral *P. violacea* collected in Australia [4], 68 interesting secondary metabolites, including 20 cembranes (29.41%), 39 briaranes (57.35%), eight briarellins (11.76%), and one secosterol (1.47%), have been isolated from octocorals belonging to the genus *Pachyclavularia*. Many studies have reported that compounds obtained from *Pachyclavularia* spp. possess various biologic activities, such as cytotoxicity (seven cembranes, six briaranes, and one briarellin), anti-inflammatory activity (three briaranes), and ichthyotoxicity (one briarane). It is interesting to note that all compounds from *Pachyclavularia* spp. reported as having been isolated between 1979 and 2014 were collected from octocorals distributed in the Indo-Pacific Ocean. The briarane-type natural products act as a chemical marker of octocorals belonging to the family Briareidae. Up to date, 379 briaranes [35–40], 13 eunicellins, 34 asbestinane, one cembrane, and one pyranone [4], have been isolated from the octocorals belonging to the family Briareidae, including the genera *Briareum* and *Erythropodium*. As more than 50% of the compounds obtained from the *Pachyclavularia* genus are briarane-type diterpenoids, we support that the taxonomic position of the *Pachyclavularia* genus should be readjusted and placed under the family Briareidae. Based on above findings, these results suggest that continuing investigation of new terpenoid analogues with the potential bioactivities from this marine organism are worthwhile for further development. The octocoral *Pachyclavularia violacea* had been transplanted to culturing tanks located in the National Museum of Marine Biology and Aquarium, Taiwan, for extraction of additional natural products to establish a stable supply of bioactive material.

Acknowledgments: This research was supported by grants from the National Museum of Marine Biology and Aquarium; the National Dong Hwa University; the National Sun Yat-sen University; and the Ministry of Science and Technology (grant nos. MOST 106-2320-B-291-001-MY3 and 104-2320-B-291-001-MY3), Taiwan, awarded to Ping-Jyun Sung.

Author Contributions: Yu-Chia Chang contributed in terms of writing the manuscript. Jyh-Horng Sheu, Yang-Chang Wu, and Ping-Jyun Sung conceived and designed the format of the manuscript. All the authors contributed in terms of critical reading and discussion of the manuscript.

Conflicts of Interest: The authors declare no conflicts of interest.

References

1. Samimi-Namin, K.; van Ofwegen, L.P. Overview of the genus *Briareum* (Cnidaria, Octocorallia, Briareidae) in the Indo-Pacific, with the description of a new species. *ZooKeys* **2016**, *557*, 1–44. [CrossRef] [PubMed]

2. Bayer, F.M. Key to the genera of octocorallia exclusive of Pennatulacea (Coelenterata: Anthozoa), with diagnoses of new taxa. *Proc. Biol. Soc. Wash.* **1981**, *94*, 902–947.

3. Bowden, B.F.; Coll, J.C.; Mitchell, S.J.; Raston, C.L.; Stokie, G.J.; White, A.H. Studies of Australian soft corals. XV. The structure of pachyclavulariadiol, a novel furano-diterpene from *Pachyclavularia violacea*. *Aust. J. Chem.* **1979**, *32*, 2265–2274. [CrossRef]

4. Sung, P.-J.; Chen, M.-C. The heterocyclic natural products of gorgonian corals of genus *Briareum* exclusive of briarane-type diterpenoids. *Heterocycles* **2002**, *57*, 1705–1715. [CrossRef]

5. Inman, W.; Crews, P. The structure and conformational properties of a cembranolide diterpene from *Clavularia violacea*. *J. Org. Chem.* **1989**, *54*, 2526–2529. [CrossRef]

6. Sheu, J.-H.; Wang, G.-H.; Sung, P.-J.; Duh, C.-Y.; Chiang, M.Y. Pachyclavulariolides G–L and secopachyclavulariaenone A, seven novel diterpenoids from the soft coral *Pachyclavularia violacea*. *Tetrahedron* **2001**, *57*, 7639–7648. [CrossRef]

7. Xu, L.; Patrick, B.O.; Roberge, M.; Allen, T.; van Ofwegen, L.; Andersen, R.J. New diterpenoids from the octocoral *Pachyclavularia violacea* collected in Papua New Guinea. *Tetrahedron* **2000**, *56*, 9031–9037. [CrossRef]

8. Sheu, J.-H.; Wang, G.-H.; Duh, C.-Y.; Soong, K. Pachyclavulariolides M–R, six novel diterpenoids from a Taiwanese soft coral *Pachyclavularia violacea*. *J. Nat. Prod.* **2003**, *66*, 662–666. [CrossRef] [PubMed]

9. Duh, C.-Y.; El-Gamal, A.A.H.; Chu, C.-J.; Wang, S.-K.; Dai, C.-F. New cytotoxic constituents from the Formosan soft corals *Clavularia viridis* and *Clavularia violacea*. *J. Nat. Prod.* **2002**, *65*, 1535–1539. [CrossRef] [PubMed]

10. Chang, Y.-C.; Huang, I.-C.; Chiang, M.Y.-N.; Hwang, T.-L.; Kung, T.-H.; Lin, C.-S.; Sheu, J.-H.; Sung, P.-J. Briaviodiol A, a new cembranoid from a soft coral *Briareum violacea*. *Chem. Pharm. Bull.* **2010**, *58*, 1666–1668. [CrossRef] [PubMed]

11. Uchio, Y.; Fukazawa, Y.; Bowden, B.F.; Coll, J.C. New diterpenes from an Australian *Pachyclavularia* species (Coelenterata, Anthozoa, Octocorallia). *Tennen Yuki Kagobutsu Toronkai Koen Yoshishu* **1989**, *31*, 548–553.

12. Cardellina, J.H., II; James, T.R., Jr.; Chen, M.H.M.; Clardy, J. Structure of brianthein W, from the soft coral *Briareum polyanthes*. *J. Org. Chem.* **1984**, *49*, 3398–3399. [CrossRef]

13. Pordesimo, E.O.; Schmitz, F.J.; Ciereszko, L.S.; Hossain, M.B.; van der Helm, D. New briarein diterpenes from the Caribbean gorgonians *Erythropodium caribaeorum* and *Briareum* sp. *J. Org. Chem.* **1991**, *56*, 2344–2357. [CrossRef]

14. Bowden, B.F.; Coll, J.C.; König, G.M. Studies of Australian soft corals. XLVIII. New briaran diterpenoids from the gorgonian coral *Junceella gemmacea*. *Aust. J. Chem.* **1990**, *43*, 151–159. [CrossRef]

15. Sheu, J.-H.; Sung, P.-J.; Huang, L.-H.; Lee, S.-F.; Wu, T.; Chang, B.-Y.; Duh, C.-Y.; Fang, L.-S.; Soong, K.; Lee, T.-J. New cytotoxic briaran diterpenes from the Formosan gorgonian *Briareum* sp. *J. Nat. Prod.* **1996**, *59*, 935–938. [CrossRef] [PubMed]

16. Wratten, S.J.; Faulkner, D.J. Some diterpenes from the sea pen *Stylatula* sp. *Tetrahedron* **1979**, *35*, 1907–1912. [CrossRef]

17. Iwasaki, J.; Ito, H.; Aoyagi, M.; Sato, Y.; Iguchi, K. Briarane-type diterpenoids from the Okinawan soft coral *Pachyclavularia violacea*. *J. Nat. Prod.* **2006**, *69*, 2–6. [CrossRef] [PubMed]

18. Ito, H.; Iwasaki, J.; Sato, Y.; Aoyagi, M.; Iguchi, K.; Yamori, T. Marine diterpenoids with a briarane skeleton from the Okinawan soft coral *Pachyclavularia violacea*. *Chem. Pharm. Bull.* **2007**, *55*, 1671–1676. [CrossRef] [PubMed]

19. Iwasaki, J.; Ito, H.; Nakamura, M.; Iguchi, K. A synthetic study of briarane-type marine diterpenoid, pachyclavulide B. *Tetrahedron Lett.* **2006**, *47*, 1483–1486. [CrossRef]
20. Ishiyama, H.; Okubo, T.; Yasuda, T.; Takahashi, Y.; Iguchi, K.; Kobayashi, J. Brianodins A–D, briarane-type diterpenoids from soft coral *Pachyclavularia* sp. *J. Nat. Prod.* **2008**, *71*, 633–636. [CrossRef] [PubMed]
21. Iwagawa, T.; Takayama, K.; Okamura, H.; Nakatani, M.; Doe, M.; Takemura, K.; Shiro, M. Cytotoxic briarane diterpenes from a gorgonacean *Briareum* sp. *Heterocycles* **1999**, *51*, 2619–2625. [CrossRef]
22. Iwagawa, T.; Hirose, T.; Takayama, K.; Okamura, H.; Nakatani, M.; Doe, M.; Takemura, K. Violides N–P, new briarane diterpenes from a gorgonacean *Briareum* sp. *Heterocycles* **2000**, *53*, 1789–1792. [CrossRef]
23. Sung, P.-J.; Su, J.-H.; Duh, C.-Y.; Chiang, M.Y.; Sheu, J.-H. Briaexcavatolides K–N, new briarane diterpenes from the gorgonian *Briareum excavatum*. *J. Nat. Prod.* **2001**, *64*, 318–323. [CrossRef] [PubMed]
24. Sung, P.-J.; Hu, W.-P.; Wu, S.-L.; Su, J.-H.; Fang, L.-S.; Wang, J.-J.; Sheu, J.-H. Briaexcavatolides X–Z, three new briarane-related derivatives from the gorgonian coral *Briareum excavatum*. *Tetrahedron* **2004**, *60*, 8975–8979. [CrossRef]
25. Iwagawa, T.; Babazono, K.; Nakatani, M.; Doe, M.; Morimoto, Y.; Takemura, K. Briarane diterpenes from a gorgonian *Briareum* sp. *Heterocycles* **2005**, *65*, 607–617. [CrossRef]
26. Sung, P.-J.; Su, Y.-D.; Li, G.-Y.; Chiang, M.Y.; Lin, M.-R.; Huang, I.-C.; Li, J.-J.; Fang, L.-S.; Wang, W.-H. Excavatoids A–D, new polyoxygenated briaranes from the octocoral *Briareum excavatum*. *Tetrahedron* **2009**, *65*, 6918–6924. [CrossRef]
27. Groweiss, A.; Look, S.A.; Fenical, W. Solenolides, new antiinflammatory and antiviral diterpenoids from a marine octocoral of the genus *Solenopodium*. *J. Org. Chem.* **1988**, *53*, 2401–2406. [CrossRef]
28. Sheu, J.-H.; Sung, P.-J.; Cheng, M.-C.; Liu, H.-Y.; Fang, L.-S.; Duh, C.-Y.; Chiang, M.Y. Novel cytotoxic diterpenes, excavatolides A–E, isolated from the Formosan gorgonian *Briareum excavatum*. *J. Nat. Prod.* **1998**, *61*, 602–608. [CrossRef] [PubMed]
29. Sheu, J.-H.; Sung, P.-J.; Su, J.-H.; Liu, H.-Y.; Duh, C.-Y.; Chiang, M.Y. Briaexcavatolides A–J, new diterpenes from the gorgonian *Briareum excavatum*. *Tetrahedron* **1999**, *55*, 14555–14564. [CrossRef]
30. Liaw, C.-C.; Cheng, Y.-B.; Lin, Y.-S.; Kuo, Y.-H.; Hwang, T.-L.; Shen, Y.-C. New briarane diterpenoids from Taiwanese soft coral *Briareum violacea*. *Mar. Drugs* **2014**, *12*, 4677–4692. [CrossRef] [PubMed]
31. Cheng, J.-F.; Yamamura, S.; Terada, Y. Stereochemistry of the brianolide acetate (=solenolide D) by the molecular mechanics calculations. *Tetrahedron Lett.* **1992**, *33*, 101–104. [CrossRef]
32. Wang, G.-H.; Sheu, J.-H.; Chiang, M.Y.; Lee, T.-J. Pachyclavulariaenones A–C, three novel diterpenoids from the soft coral *Pachyclavularia violacea*. *Tetrahedron Lett.* **2001**, *42*, 2333–2336. [CrossRef]
33. Wang, G.-H.; Sheu, J.-H.; Duh, C.-Y.; Chiang, M.Y. Pachyclavulariaenones D–G, new diterpenoids from the soft coral *Pachyclavularia violacea*. *J. Nat. Prod.* **2002**, *65*, 1475–1478. [CrossRef] [PubMed]
34. Anta, C.; González, N.; Rodríguez, J.; Jiménez, C. A new secosterol from the Indonesian octocoral *Pachyclavularia violacea*. *J. Nat. Prod.* **2002**, *65*, 1357–1359. [CrossRef] [PubMed]
35. Sung, P.-J.; Sheu, J.-H.; Xu, J.-P. Survey of briarane-type diterpenoids of marine origin. *Heterocycles* **2002**, *57*, 535–579. [CrossRef]
36. Sung, P.-J.; Chang, P.-J.; Fang, L.-S.; Sheu, J.-H.; Chen, W.-C.; Chen, Y.-P.; Lin, M.-R. Survey of briarane-type diterpenoids-Part II. *Heterocycles* **2005**, *65*, 195–204. [CrossRef]
37. Sung, P.-J.; Sheu, J.-H.; Wang, W.-H.; Fang, L.-S.; Chung, H.-M.; Pai, C.-H.; Su, Y.-D.; Tsai, W.-T.; Chen, B.-Y.; Lin, M.-R.; et al. Survey of briarane-type diterpenoids-Part III. *Heterocycles* **2008**, *75*, 2627–2648. [CrossRef]
38. Sung, P.-J.; Su, J.-H.; Wang, W.-H.; Sheu, J.-H.; Fang, L.-S.; Wu, Y.-C.; Chen, Y.-H.; Chung, H.-M.; Su, Y.-D.; Chang, Y.-C. Survey of briarane-type diterpenoids-Part IV. *Heterocycles* **2011**, *83*, 1241–1258. [CrossRef]
39. Sheu, J.-H.; Chen, Y.-H.; Chen, Y.-H.; Su, Y.-D.; Chang, Y.-C.; Su, J.-H.; Weng, C.-F.; Lee, C.-H.; Fang, L.-S.; Wang, W.-H.; et al. Briarane diterpenoids isolated from gorgonian corals between 2011 and 2013. *Mar. Drugs* **2014**, *12*, 2164–2181. [CrossRef] [PubMed]
40. Su, Y.-D.; Su, J.-H.; Hwang, T.-L.; Wen, Z.-H.; Sheu, J.-H.; Wu, Y.-C.; Sung, P.-J. Briarane diterpenoids isolated from octocorals between 2014 and 2016. *Mar. Drugs* **2017**, *15*, 44. [CrossRef] [PubMed]

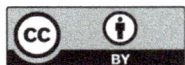

marine drugs

MDPI

Article

The Bioactive Extract of *Pinnigorgia* sp. Induces Apoptosis of Hepatic Stellate Cells via ROS-ERK/JNK-Caspase-3 Signaling

Liang-Mou Kuo [1,2,†], Po-Jen Chen [3,4,†], Ping-Jyun Sung [5,6,7,8,9], Yu-Chia Chang [6,10], Chun-Ting Ho [3], Yi-Hsiu Wu [3] and Tsong-Long Hwang [3,4,11,12,*]

[1] Graduate Institute of Clinical Medical Sciences, College of Medicine, Chang Gung University, Taoyuan 333, Taiwan; kuo33410@yahoo.com.tw
[2] Department of General Surgery, Chang Gung Memorial Hospital, Chiayi 613, Taiwan
[3] Graduate Institute of Natural Products, College of Medicine, Chang Gung University, Taoyuan 333, Taiwan; litlep@hotmail.com (P.-J.C.); Tsudanyer@hotmail.com (C.-T.H.); modemtw@gmail.com (Y.-H.W.)
[4] Chinese Herbal Medicine Research Team, Healthy Aging Research Center, Chang Gung University, Taoyuan 333, Taiwan
[5] Graduate Institute of Marine Biology, National Dong Hwa University, Pingtung 944, Taiwan; pjsung@nmmba.gov.tw
[6] National Museum of Marine Biology and Aquarium, Pingtung 944, Taiwan; jay0404@gmail.com
[7] Chinese Medicine Research and Development Center, China Medical University Hospital, Taichung 404, Taiwan
[8] Graduate Institute of Natural Products, Kaohsiung Medical University, Kaohsiung 807, Taiwan
[9] Department of Marine Biotechnology and Resources, National Sun Yat-sen University, Kaohsiung 804, Taiwan
[10] Doctoral Degree Program in Marine Biotechnology, National Sun Yat-sen University & Academia Sinica, Kaohsiung 804, Taiwan
[11] Research Center for Chinese Herbal Medicine, Research Center for Food and Cosmetic Safety, Graduate Institute of Health Industry Technology, College of Human Ecology, Chang Gung University of Science and Technology, Taoyuan 333, Taiwan
[12] Department of Anaesthesiology, Chang Gung Memorial Hospital, Taoyuan 333, Taiwan
*   Correspondence: htl@mail.cgu.edu.tw; Tel.: +886-32-118-800
†   These authors contributed equally to this work.

Received: 4 December 2017; Accepted: 6 January 2018; Published: 9 January 2018

Abstract: The activation of hepatic stellate cells (HSCs) is a significant phenomenon during the pathogenesis of liver disorders, including liver cirrhosis and fibrosis. Here, we identified that the extract from a gorgonian coral *Pinnigorgia* sp. (Pin) induced apoptosis of HSC-T6 cells. Pin inhibited the viability of HSC-T6 cells and increased their subG1 population, DNA fragmentation, caspase-3 activation, and reactive oxygen species (ROS) production in a concentration-dependent manner. The Pin-induced ROS generation and apoptotic effects were significantly reversed by a thiol antioxidant, *N*-acetylcysteine (NAC). Additionally, Pin induced ERK/JNK phosphorylation and pharmacological inhibition of ERK/JNK rescued the Pin-induced cell death. Pin-activated ERK/JNK were significantly reduced after the administration of NAC; however, the inhibition of ERK/JNK failed to change the Pin-induced ROS production. Similarly, pinnigorgiol A, a pure compound isolated from Pin, elicited ROS production and apoptosis in HSC-T6 cells. The pinnigorgiol A-induced apoptosis was retrained by NAC. Together, it appears that Pin leads to apoptosis in HSC-T6 cells through ROS-mediated ERK/JNK signaling and caspase-3 activation. Pinnigorgiol A serves as a bioactive compound of Pin and may exhibit therapeutic potential by clearance of HSCs.

Keywords: hepatic stellate cells; *Pinnigorgia* sp.; ROS; apoptosis; caspase-3; MAPK

1. Introduction

Hepatic fibrosis is an early significant lesion in chronic liver diseases such as liver cirrhosis and hepatocellular carcinoma. The excessive activation and proliferation of hepatic stellate cells (HSCs) gives rise to pro-inflammatory growth factors and extracellular matrix proteins during the pathogenesis of hepatic fibrosis, initiating matrix deposition in the liver [1–3]. Emerging evidences reveal that the restriction of activated HSCs is a potential strategy for hepatic fibrosis therapy via repressing proliferation or inducing apoptosis of HSCs [4–7]. So far, natural products derived from marine organisms display various potential pharmacological activities, including those applicable in liver disorder [8–10]. It is desirable to develop novel and useful marine natural products as better remedial strategies for hepatic disease through reversing the activated HSCs back to their quiescent status.

The *Pinnigorgia* sp. (Figure 1A) was first isolated and identified as in Taiwan [11]. Taxonomically, gorgonian coral *Pinnigorgia* sp. belongs to the animal kingdom (Kingdom Animalia), Cnidaria (Phylum Cnidaria), Anthozoa (Class Anthozoa), Octocorals subclass (Subclass Octocorallia), Gorgonian head (Order Gorgonacea), Holaxonia suborder, Family Gorgoniidae. Recently, various natural compounds from a gorgonian coral *Pinnigorgia* sp. have been shown to exhibit anti-inflammatory potential in human neutrophils [11–15]. In addition, the coralline extract from *Pinnigorgia* sp. (Pin) reduces the survival rate of HSCs [11,16], although the underlying mechanisms are still elusive. Therefore, it can be suggested that Pin may possess potential application to attenuate liver fibrosis via retraining the HSCs activation.

The aim of this study was to uncover the pharmacological mechanism of Pin-inhibited cell viability in a rat HSC cell line, HSC-T6 cells. During proliferation and activation of HSCs, intracellular redox homeostasis tightly controls the cell viability. Intracellular glutathione (GSH) level is an important factor to modulate redox balance [17]. GSH depletion induces reactive oxygen species (ROS) accumulation, leading to caspase-3-dependent apoptosis in HSCs [18–20]. Moreover, mitogen-activated protein kinases (MAPKs) signaling is also involved in redox homeostasis and apoptosis in HSCs [20–23].

In the present study, we found that the Pin-repressed cell viability in HSCs was dependent on caspase-3-, ROS-, and ERK/JNK-mediated apoptosis. Pin-induced ERK/JNK activation occurred through ROS production. The caspase-3 inhibitor, thiol antioxidants, and ERK/JNK inhibitors significantly abolished the Pin-induced cell death in HSCs. Moreover, pinnigorgiol A served as a bioactive compound of Pin that triggered the apoptosis and ROS production in HSCs. Our findings suggest that marine natural products from gorgonian coral including Pin and pinnigorgiol A exhibit therapeutic potentials by clearance of HSCs.

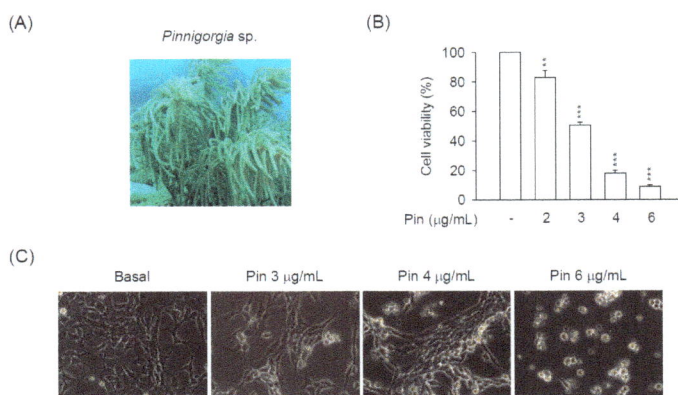

Figure 1. *Cont.*

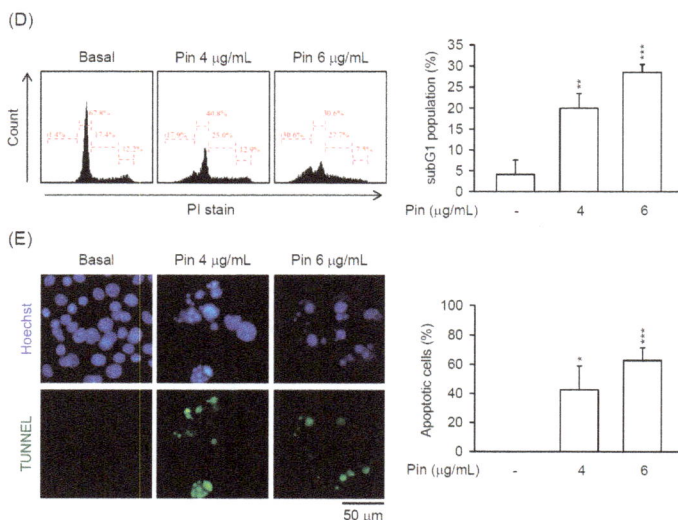

Figure 1. Pin elicits apoptosis in hepatic stellate cells (HSCs). HSC-T6 cells were treated with Pin (0–6 μg/mL) for 24 h. (**A**) Gorgonian coral *Pinnigorgia* sp.; (**B**) Cytotoxicity assay was monitored spectrophotometrically at 450 nm; (**C**) Cell retraction, bubbling, and apoptotic bodies were observed using microscopy; (**D**) SubG1 population was examined by propidium iodide (PI) staining and flow cytometry; (**E**) The Pin-induced apoptosis of HSC-T6 cells was determined by terminal deoxynucleotidyl transferase dUTP nick end labeling (TUNEL) assay (green). Hoechst 33,342 (blue) was used to visualize the cell nucleus. All data are expressed as the mean ± S.E.M. (*n* = 3). * *p* < 0.05, ** *p* < 0.01, *** *p* < 0.001 compared with the basal.

2. Results

2.1. Pin Exhibits Caspase-3-Dependent Apoptosis in HSC-T6 Cells

Recently, the extract from a gorgonian coral *Pinnigorgia* sp. (Pin) was isolated and found to suppress the cell viability of rat HSC-T6 cells [11]. However, the pharmacological mechanism of Pin-induced suppression of HSC-T6 cell viability is still undiscovered. Here, we studied the detailed mechanism of Pin-inhibited viability in HSCs. Pin inhibited the cell viability of HSC-T6 cells in a concentration-dependent manner (2–6 μg/mL) (Figure 1B). To monitor the Pin-induced cell death in HSC-T6 cells, we observed the changes in cellular morphology. Pin (3–6 μg/mL) gradually led to the apoptotic changes of HSC-T6 cells, including cell shrinkage and the formation of membrane blebs, apoptotic body, and cell debris (Figure 1C). To further determine the apoptotic features, flow cytometry and terminal deoxynucleotidyl transferase (TdT) dUTP nick-end labeling (TUNEL) staining were assayed. Pin (4 and 6 μg/mL) apparently increased the subG1 population, which was as an indicator of apoptosis. Also, Pin (4 and 6 μg/mL) induced DNA fragmentation in HSC-T6 cells (Figure 1D,E).

Caspase-3 plays a central role in apoptotic responses. As shown in the results, the expression of cleaved caspase-3 was significantly increased in Pin (6 μg/mL)-treated HSC-T6 cells during 9–24 h (Figure 2A). Moreover, the Pin-inhibited cell viability in HSC-T6 cells was blocked by pre-treatment of the general caspase inhibitor, Z-VAD-FMK, or the specific caspase-3 inhibitor, Z-DEVD-FMK (Figure 2B), suggesting that Pin-induced apoptosis in HSC-T6 cells occurs through caspase-3-dependent pathway.

(A)

(B)

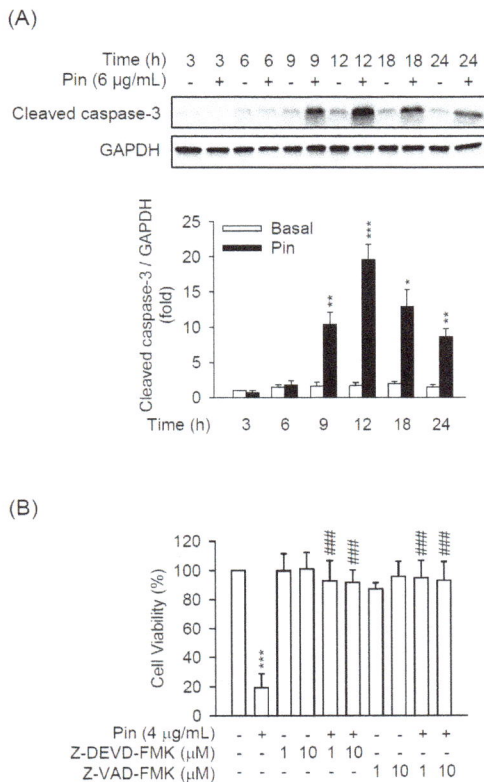

Figure 2. Pin-induced apoptosis is dependent on caspase-3 activation in HSCs. (**A**) HSC-T6 cells were treated with Pin (6 μg/mL) for 3–24 h. Cleaved caspase-3 and glyceraldehyde-3-phosphate dehydrogenase (GAPDH) were analyzed by immunoblot analysis using antibodies against cleaved caspase-3 or GAPDH. Quantitation of the cleaved caspase-3/GAPDH ratio is shown; (**B**) HSC-T6 cells were pretreated with Z-DEVD-FMK (caspase-3 inhibitor) or Z-VAD-FMK (general caspase inhibitor) for 1 h. Subsequently, HSC-T6 was incubated with Pin (4 μg/mL) for 24 h. The cytotoxicity assay was monitored spectrophotometrically at 450 nm. All data are expressed as the mean ± S.E.M. (n = 3). * $p < 0.05$, ** $p < 0.01$, *** $p < 0.001$ compared with the basal; ### $p < 0.001$ compared with the Pin alone.

2.2. Pin-Induced Apoptosis Is Dependent on Intracellular ROS Production in HSC-T6 Cells

Until now, GSH depletion-induced ROS accumulation is known to cause caspase-3-dependent apoptosis in HSCs [18,19]. To investigate whether Pin causes oxidative stress in HSCs, the intracellular ROS production was determined. Pin induced ROS production in HSC-T6 cells in a dose-dependent (3–6 μg/mL) manner (Figure 3A). Furthermore, the thiol-antioxidant, NAC, inhibited the Pin-induced ROS generation in HSC-T6 cells (Figure 3B). Importantly, both NAC and a permeable membrane derivative of GSH, glutathione monoethyl ester (GSH-MEE), apparently attenuated the Pin-induced caspase-3 activation, cell death, and DNA fragmentation in HSC-T6 cells (Figures 3C,D and S1), suggesting that the Pin-induced ROS production is a cause of cell death in HSC-T6 cells.

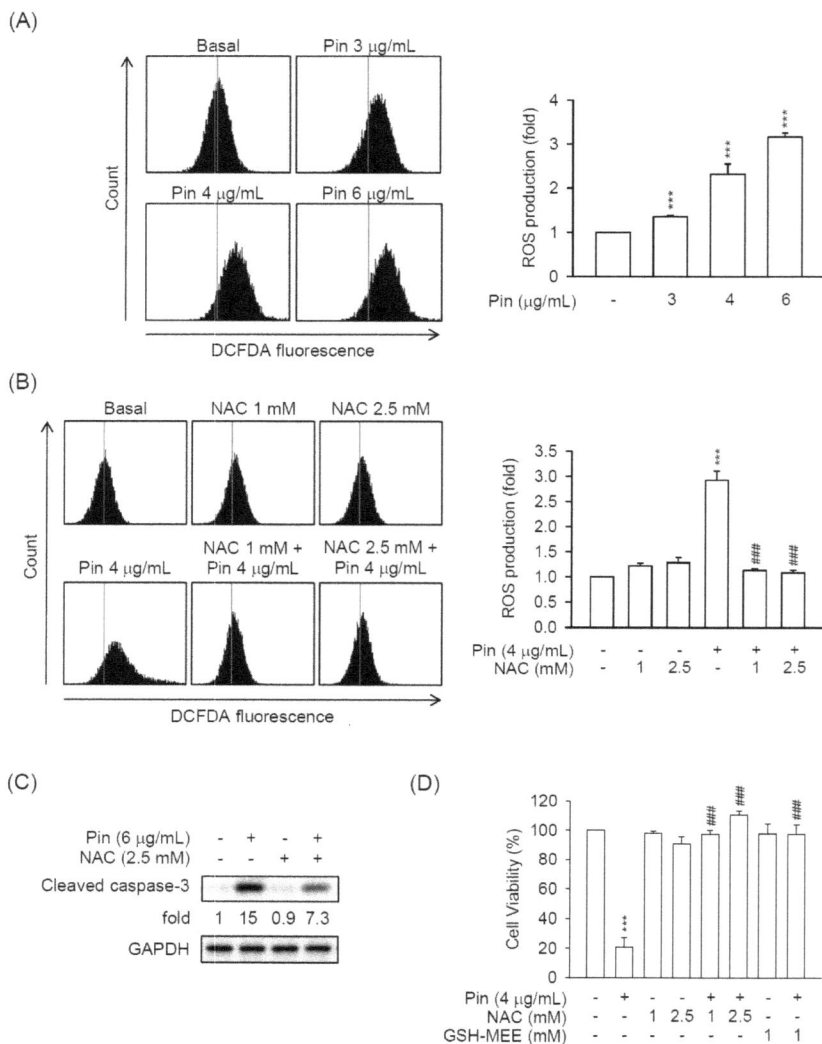

Figure 3. Pin-induced apoptosis relies on intracellular reactive oxygen species (ROS) production in HSCs. (**A**) HSC-T6 cells were treated with Pin (3–6 μg/mL) for 6 h. Intracellular ROS was determined by 2′,7′-dichlorofluorescein diacetate (DCFDA) assay using flow cytometry; (**B**) HSC-T6 cells were pretreated with *N*-acetylcysteine (NAC; 1 and 2.5 mM for 1 h) before the addition of Pin (4 μg/mL for 6 h). Intracellular ROS was determined by DCFDA assay using flow cytometry; (**C**) HSC-T6 cells were pretreated with NAC (2.5 mM) for 1 h and then exposed to Pin (6 μg/mL) for 12 h. Cleaved caspase-3 and GAPDH was analyzed by immunoblot analysis using antibodies against cleaved caspase-3 or GAPDH; (**D**) HSC-T6 cells were pretreated with NAC (1 and 2.5 mM) or glutathione reduced ethyl ester (GSH-MEE) (1 mM) for 1 h and then exposed to Pin (4 μg/mL) for 24 h. The cytotoxicity assay was monitored spectrophotometrically at 450 nm. All data are expressed as the mean ± S.E.M. ($n = 3$). *** $p < 0.001$ compared with the basal. ### $p < 0.001$ compared with the Pin alone.

2.3. Pin-Induced Cell Death of HSC-T6 Cells Is through ERK and JNK Pathway

The significance of MAPKs pathway in cell growth and apoptosis has been well established [24]. Therefore, we next examined whether MAPKs is involved in the Pin-induced apoptosis in HSC-T6 cells. Pin (6 µg/mL) significantly induced the phosphorylation of ERK and JNK but not p38 MAPK in HSC-T6 cells for 3–12 h (Figure S2A). In addition, Pin led to ERK and JNK activation in HSC-T6 cells in a dose-dependent manner. The pharmacological inhibitors of JNK (SP600125) and ERK (PD98059) completely blocked the Pin-repressed cell viability in HSC-T6 cells (Figure 4), suggesting the critical role of ERK and JNK activation in Pin-induced apoptosis in HSCs. In agreement with the inactivation of p38 MAPK in Pin-treated HSC-T6 cells, the inhibitors of p38 (SB202190 and 203580) failed to restrict the Pin-induced cell death (Figure S2B).

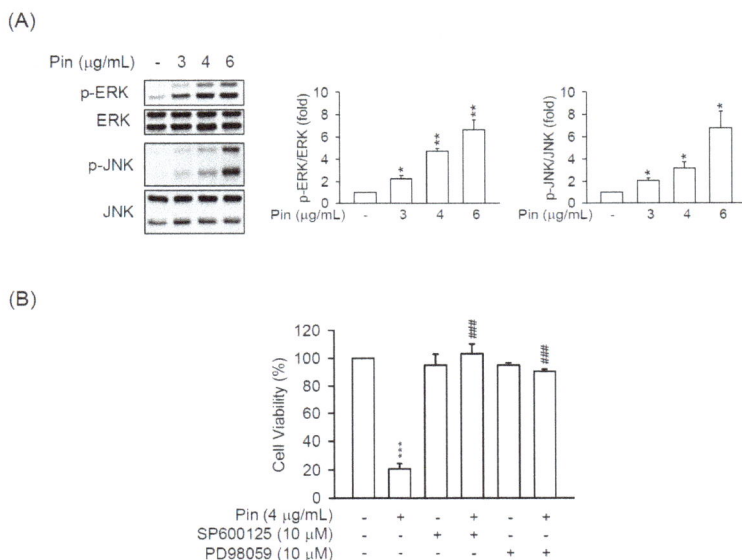

Figure 4. Pin-induced apoptosis is mediated through JNK and ERK pathway in HSCs. (**A**) HSC-T6 cells were treated with Pin (3–6 µg/mL) for 6 h. Phosphorylation of ERK and JNK were analyzed by immunoblot analysis using antibodies against p-JNK or p-ERK. Quantitation of the p-JNK/JNK and p-ERK/ERK ratio was shown; (**B**) HSC-T6 cells were pretreated with SP600125 (JNK inhibitor; 10 µM) or PD98059 (ERK inhibitor; 10 µM) for 1 h and then exposure to Pin (4 µg/mL) for 24 h. Cytotoxicity assay was monitored spectrophotometrically at 450 nm. All data are expressed as the mean ± S.E.M. ($n = 3$). * $p < 0.05$, ** $p < 0.01$, *** $p < 0.001$ compared with the basal. ### $p < 0.001$ compared with the Pin alone.

2.4. Pin-Activated ERK and JNK Pathway Act as Downstream Signals of ROS Production in HSC-T6 Cells

It has been documented that ERK may be an upstream regulator of ROS-induced apoptosis [25], however, different studies have reported conflicting findings [26]. To clarify the relationship between ROS and ERK/JNK in Pin-treated HSC-T6 cells, the HSC-T6 cells were pre-treated with inhibitors of ERK/JNK or thiol-antioxidant to examine it. As shown in the results, NAC evidently restrained the Pin-induced ERK and JNK activation in HSC-T6 cells (Figure 5A). In contrast, the inhibitors of JNK (SP600125) and ERK (PD98059) failed to alter Pin-induced ROS production in HSC-T6 cells (Figure 5B). Taken together, we propose that Pin stimulates the ROS production and subsequently activates ERK/JNK signaling leading to caspase-3-dependent cell death in HSC-T6 cells.

(A)

(B)

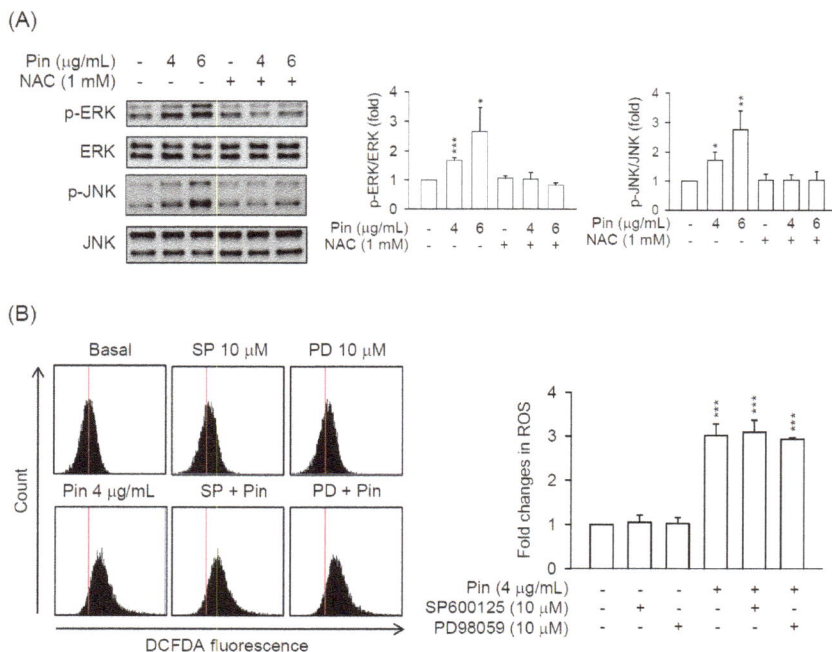

Figure 5. Pin-activated ERK and JNK signaling is triggered by ROS production in HSCs. (**A**) HSC-T6 cells were pretreated with or without NAC (1 mM) for 1 h and then exposed to Pin (4 or 6 μg/mL) for 6 h. Phosphorylation of ERK and JNK were analyzed by immunoblot analysis using antibodies against p-JNK or p-ERK. Quantitation of the p-JNK/JNK and p-ERK/ERK ratio was shown; (**B**) HSC-T6 cells were pretreated with SP600125 (JNK inhibitor; 10 μM) or PD98059 (ERK inhibitor; 10 μM) for 1 h and then exposed to Pin (4 μg/mL) for 6 h. Intracellular ROS was determined by DCFDA assay using flow cytometry. All data are expressed as the mean ± S.E.M. (*n* = 3). * *p* < 0.05, ** *p* < 0.01, *** *p* < 0.001 compared with the basal.

2.5. Pinnigorgiol a Serves as a Bioactive Component of Pin to Trigger the ROS-Dependent Apoptosis in HSC-T6 Cells

Three novel 9,11-secosterols, pinnigorgiol A–C, were isolated from Pin to test the viability of HSC-T6 cells. Among them, pinnigorgiol A and B displayed inhibitory effect on the cell viability with an IC$_{50}$ value of 5.77 ± 0.27 and 7.89 ± 0.52 μM, respectively, but pinnigorgiol C had no effect on cell viability [16]. Pinnigorgiol A (Figure 6A) exhibited the maximum inhibitory effect on the cell viability of HSC-T6 cells; however, the pharmacological mechanism is still unknown. As shown in Figure 6B, pinnigorgiol A (1–10 μM) inhibited the cell viability of HSC-T6 cells in a dose-dependent manner. Pinnigorgiol B (3–10 μM) also dose-dependently repressed the cell viability of HSC-T6 cells (Figure S3); however, the inhibitory effect was weaker than pinnigorgiol A. Further, pinnigorgiol A induced ROS production and DNA fragmentation in HSC-T6 cells. Furthermore, the pinnigorgiol A-induced apoptotic effect and cell death were significantly attenuated by the thio-antioxidant NAC in HSC-T6 cells (Figure 6C–E), suggesting that the cytotoxic effect of Pin and pinnigorgiol A is comparable in HSCs. In summary, we propose that pinnigorgiol A may be a representative bioactive component of Pin that elicits apoptosis in HSCs through ROS-ERK/JNK-caspase-3 signal pathway and may offer a possible medical application in liver pathogenesis.

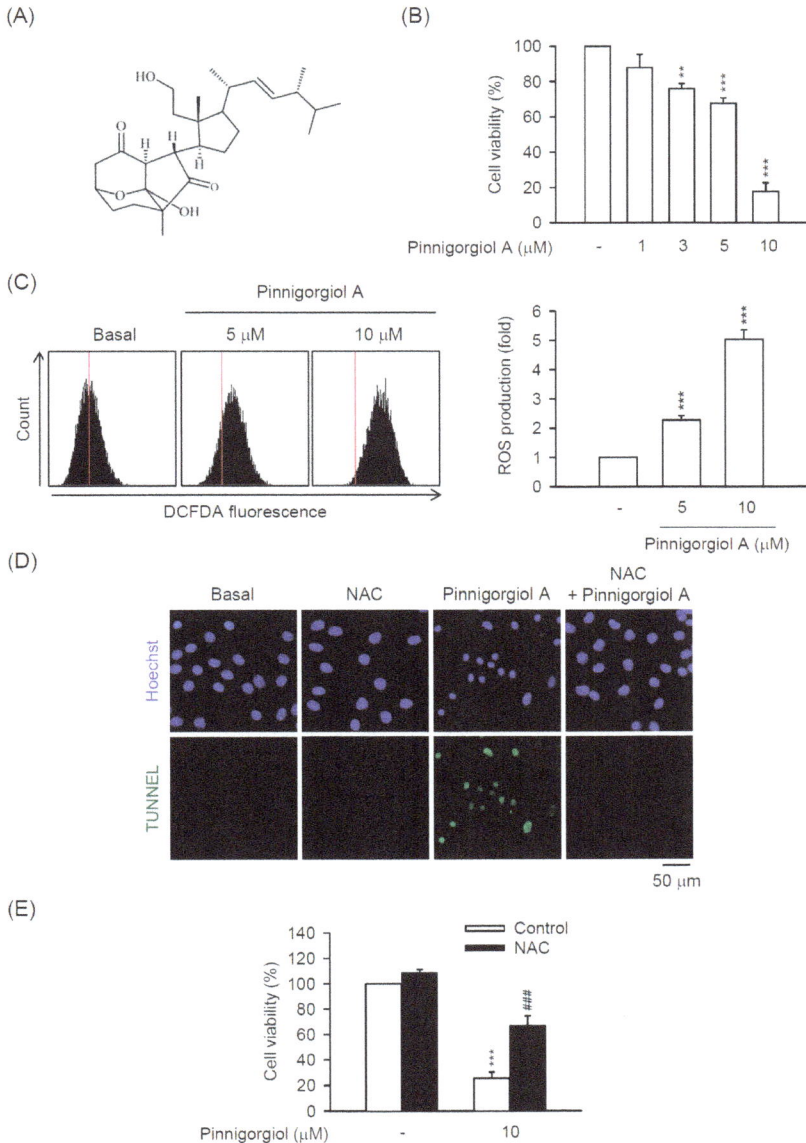

Figure 6. Pinnigorgiol A exhibits ROS-dependent apoptosis in HSCs. (**A**) Chemical structure of pinnigorgiol A; (**B**) HSC-T6 cells were treated with pinnigorgiol A (1–10 µM) for 24 h. Cytotoxicity assay was monitored spectrophotometrically at 450 nm; (**C**) HSC-T6 cells were treated with pinnigorgiol A (5 or 10 µM) for 6 h. Intracellular ROS was determined by DCFDA assay and flow cytometry; (**D**) HSC-T6 cells were treated with pinnigorgiol A (10 µM) for 12 h. Apoptotic effect of pinnigorgiol A was determined by TUNEL assay (green). Hoechst 33,342 (blue) was used to visualize the cell nucleus; (**E**) HSC-T6 cells were pretreated with NAC (2.5 mM) for 1 h and then incubated with pinnigorgiol A (10 µM) for 24 h. Cytotoxicity assay was monitored spectrophotometrically at 450 nm. All data are expressed as the mean ± S.E.M. ($n = 3$). ** $p < 0.01$; *** $p < 0.001$ compared with the basal. ### $p < 0.001$ compared with the pinnigorgiol A alone.

3. Discussion

The activation of HSCs is one of the major contributors to hepatic fibrosis. Emerging evidences show that promoting cell death of HSCs is a potential strategy in the remission of liver fibrosis [4,5,27,28]. In the present study, our data revealed that Pin significantly induced cell apoptosis in HSCs in a concentration-dependent way. Pin significantly exhibited an inhibitory effect on the cell viability in HSC-T6 cells with apparent apoptotic changes, including cell shrinkage, chromatin condensation, and membrane blebs and apoptotic bodies formation (Figure 1). Moreover, it has been proven that DNA fragmentation usually accompanies increased sub-G1 population and activated caspase-3 in apoptotic cells [29–31]. We also found that Pin increased the sub-G1 population, DNA fragmentation, and caspase-3 activation in HSC-T6 cells (Figures 1 and 2A), suggesting that the Pin-repressed HSCs viability is dependent on caspase-3-mediated apoptosis. In agreement with this proposal, the apoptotic effects of Pin were completely reversed by Z-DEVD-FMK, a specific caspase-3 inhibitor (Figure 3B). Activation of caspase-3 has a pivotal role in the apoptotic responses. Thus, Pin stimulated the apoptotic process in HSCs through caspase-3-dependent pathway. These findings suggest a possibility of Pin to restrict HSCs activation during liver pathogenesis.

Oxidative stress can induce the execution of the apoptotic pathway and excessive ROS production will lead to aggravation of apoptosis [32–34]. So far, ROS generation has been documented to cause apoptosis in HSCs [18,20,35]. In support of this theory, intracellular ROS was increased by treatment of Pin in HSC-T6 cells that was significantly reversed by a thiol-based antioxidant, NAC (Figure 3). In addition, GSH is another intracellular antioxidant that regulates the cell viability in HSCs and GSH displays an inhibitory effect against ROS-induced apoptotic cell death [17,18]. In addition, NAC and cell-permeable GSH (GSH-MEE) significantly blocked the Pin-inhibited cell viability in HSC-T6 cells, suggesting that the Pin-induced apoptosis is based on ROS production in HSCs.

MAPKs (ERK, JNK, and p38 MAPK) are important mediators of signal transduction under oxidative stress in HSCs to control cell growth, differentiation, survival, and apoptosis [18,36–38]. In our previous study, the apoptotic effect of oridonin-induced ROS in HSC-T6 cells was not affected by specific inhibitors of p38 MAPK, JNK, and ERK, respectively [20]. However, Huang and colleagues found that the oridonin-induced apoptosis and ROS production in HepG2 cells occurred through MAPK signaling pathways [37]. Thus, the role of MAPKs in the oxidative stress-elicited HSCs apoptosis is still uncertain. As the results showed, Pin induced the phosphorylation of ERK and JNK but not p38 MAPK in HSCs (Figures 4 and S2). Pharmacological inhibitors of JNK (SP600125) and ERK (PD98059) rescued the Pin-induced cell apoptosis in HSCs, suggesting that the apoptotic effects of Pin in HSC were mediated by ERK and JNK. It has been documented that blocking the p38 MAPK by a specific inhibitor, SB203580, increased the proliferation in HSCs [39], whereas activation of p38 induced HSC apoptosis [10,40]. This may explain the selective inhibition of Pin on the activation of ERK and JNK but not p38 MAPK in HSCs, which may also serve as a means to explore the relationship between MAPKs and apoptosis in HSCs.

Three pure compounds, pinnigorgiol A-C, were isolated from Pin to decrease the viability of HSC-T6 cells at 10 μM. Among them, pinnigorgiol A displayed the maximum inhibitory effect on the cell viability with an IC_{50} value of 5.77 ± 0.27 μM [16]. In the present study, we unraveled that pinnigorgiol A-induced apoptosis of HSCs was also mediated by increasing ROS production (Figure 6), suggesting that pinnigorgiol A may be the representative bioactive compound of Pin leading to cell death in HSCs. To date, marine bioactive compounds have been characterized and have therapeutic potential to treat human disorders; however, the studies investigating their role in treating liver diseases are still limited [10]. Therefore, pinnigorgiol A may provide a therapeutic opportunity to retrain HSCs activation in liver fibrosis. Activation of HSCs is mediated by various mechanisms and some of them exhibit the therapeutic specificity for restricting HSC activation but not affecting hepatocytes [2]. In this study, the proof of whether Pin or pinnigorgiol A leads to apoptosis in hepatocytes is not carried out yet. The possible liver injuries by Pin or pinnigorgiol A still should be carefully dissected in the future.

In summary, our findings reveal an important example of how a novel coral extract from *Pinnigorgia* sp. (Pin) leads to a caspase-3-dependent apoptosis in HSCs via inducing ROS-mediated ERK/JNK signaling. Pinnigorgiol A may be a bioactive compound of Pin that possibly attenuates HSCs activation in liver fibrosis.

4. Materials and Methods

4.1. Reagents

Glutathione monoethyl ester (GSH-MEE) was purchased from Calbiochem (La Jolla, CA, USA). Z-DEVD-FMK and Z-VAD-FMK were obtained from BioVision (Mountain, PA, USA). The cell proliferation reagent WST-1 and RNase A were obtained from Roche Applied Sciences (Mannheim, Germany). Antibodies against cleaved caspase-3, phospho-ERK1/2, ERK1/2, phospho-JNK, and JNK were purchased from Cell Signaling (Beverly, MA, USA). Antibodies against phospho-p38 and p38 MAPK were obtained from Santa Cruz Biotechnology (Santa Cruz, CA, USA). The other chemicals were purchased from Sigma (St. Louis, MO, USA). The extraction and isolation of crude extract from *Pinnigorgia* sp. (Pin) and pinnigorgiol A were carried out as described previously [11,16]. The ^{1}H and ^{13}C NMR spectrum of pinnigorgiol A–C have been identified previously [16]. When Pin and pinnigorgiol A were dissolved in dimethyl sulfoxide (DMSO) (Sigma-Aldrich), the final concentration of DMSO in the cell experiments was 0.1% and did not affect the parameters measured.

4.2. Cell Culture

HSC-T6, a rat HSC cell line, was kindly provided by Professor Scott L. Friedman (Mount Sinai School of Medicine, NY, USA). HSC-T6 cells were cultured at 37 °C in Dulbecco's minimum essential medium (DMEM; Gibco, Grand Island, NY, USA) supplemented with 10% fetal bovine serum (FBS) and antibiotics (100 U/mL penicillin, 100 µg/mL streptomycin, and 2.5 µg/mL amphotericin B) in a humidified atmosphere with 5% CO_2.

4.3. Cell Viability Assay

Cell viability was measured using WST-1 assay. HSC-T6 cells were cultured in DMEM containing 0.5% FBS for 24 h. After incubation, cells were incubated with indicated concentrations of Pin or pinnigorgiol A for 24 h. Subsequently, the WST-1 reagent was added and incubated at 37 °C for 2 h. The absorbance was measured spectrophotometrically at 450 nm (Thermo Labsystems, Waltham, MA, USA).

4.4. Analysis of SubG1 Population

HSC-T6 cells were treated with Pin for 24 h and then the cells were harvested and fixed in 70% ethanol for 1 h. After that, the cells were washed with PBS twice and incubated in propidium iodide staining buffer (50 µg/mL propidium iodide, 0.1 mg/mL DNase-free RNase A, and 0.5% Triton X-100) for 30 min at 37 °C. The subG1 population was determined by measuring DNA content using flow cytometry.

4.5. Measurement of Intracellular ROS Generation

The intracellular ROS levels were examined using 2′,7′-dichlorofluorescein diacetate (DCF-DA; Sigma) reagent and analyzed by flow cytometry (BD Biosciences, San Jose, CA, USA).

4.6. Western Blotting

Cell lysates were suspended in lysis buffer (50 mM HEPES, 100 mM NaCl, 1 mM EDTA, 2 mM Na_3VO_4, 5% 2-mercaptoethanol, and 1% Triton-X-100), and then centrifuged at 14,000× *g* for 20 min at 4 °C. Proteins were separated by sodium dodecyl sulfate-polyacrylamide gel electrophoresis (SDS-PAGE) and electrophoresed onto a nitrocellulose membrane. Indicated primary antibodies and horseradish peroxidase-conjugated secondary antibodies were used to determine the protein levels using an enhanced chemiluminescence system. Signals were detected and quantified using a densitometer (UVP, Upland, CA, USA).

4.7. TUNEL Assay

The DNA fragmentation in apoptosis was detected using terminal deoxyribonucleotidyl transferase-mediated dUTP-digoxigenin nick end labeling (TUNEL) apoptosis detection kit (Roche, Mannheim, Germany). The nuclei were counterstained with DAPI. Visual images were analyzed using an OLYMPUS IX 81 microscope (Olympus, Tokyo, Japan).

4.8. Statistical Analysis

Data were expressed as the mean ± standard error of mean (SEM). Statistical comparisons were made between two groups using Student's *t*-test. A value of $p < 0.05$ was considered statistically significant.

5. Conclusions

Clearance of activated HSCs is a potential strategy to treat liver fibrosis by pharmacologically prompting apoptosis. In the present study, we found that the extract from a gorgonian coral *Pinnigorgia* sp. (Pin) led to caspase-3-dependent apoptosis in HSCs that is modulated via ROS production and subsequent ERK/JNK activation. Moreover, the Pin-derived pure compound, pinnigorgiol A, was identified as a bioactive component which elicited apoptosis and ROS production in HSCs. Altogether, we uncovered the molecular mechanisms of the marine natural products, Pin and pinnigorgiol A, and predicted their therapeutic potential eliminating HSCs in liver diseases.

Supplementary Materials: The following are available online at www.mdpi.com/1660-3397/16/1/19/s1, Figure S1. *N*-acetylcysteine (NAC) abolishes the Pin-induced apoptosis in hepatic stellate cells (HSCs), Figure S2. Pin-induced apoptosis is independent of p38 MAPK in HSCs, Figure S3. Pinnigorgiol B inhibits the cell viability of HSCs.

Acknowledgments: This research was financial supported by the grants from the Ministry of Science Technology (MOST 106-2320-B-255-003-MY3 and MOST 104-2320-B-255-004-MY3), Ministry of Education (EMRPD1G0231), and Chang Gung Memorial Hospital (CMRPG660201, CMRPG670421, CMRPG6D0081~3, CMRPF1F0011~3, CMRPF1F0061~3, and BMRP450), Taiwan. The funders had no role in study design, data collection and analysis, decision to publish, or preparation of the manuscript.

Author Contributions: L.-M.K., P.-J.C., C.-T.H. and Y.-H.W. designed, performed and analyzed experiments. P.-J.S. and Y.-C.C. provided Pin and pinnigorgiol A. P.-J.C. and T.-L.H. wrote and completed the manuscript. T.-L.H. supervised the entire study.

Conflicts of Interest: The authors declare no conflict of interest.

References

1. Yin, C.; Evason, K.J.; Asahina, K.; Stainier, D.Y. Hepatic stellate cells in liver development, regeneration, and cancer. *J. Clin. Investig.* **2013**, *123*, 1902–1910. [CrossRef] [PubMed]
2. Tsuchida, T.; Friedman, S.L. Mechanisms of hepatic stellate cell activation. *Nat. Rev. Gastroenterol. Hepatol.* **2017**, *14*, 397–411. [CrossRef] [PubMed]
3. Tacke, F.; Trautwein, C. Mechanisms of liver fibrosis resolution. *J. Hepatol.* **2015**, *63*, 1038–1039. [CrossRef] [PubMed]
4. Friedman, S.L. Evolving challenges in hepatic fibrosis. *Nat. Rev. Gastroenterol. Hepatol.* **2010**, *7*, 425–436. [CrossRef] [PubMed]
5. Huang, Y.; Deng, X.; Liang, J. Modulation of hepatic stellate cells and reversibility of hepatic fibrosis. *Exp. Cell Res.* **2017**, *352*, 420–426. [CrossRef] [PubMed]
6. Zhang, C.Y.; Yuan, W.G.; He, P.; Lei, J.H.; Wang, C.X. Liver fibrosis and hepatic stellate cells: Etiology, pathological hallmarks and therapeutic targets. *World J. Gastroenterol.* **2016**, *22*, 10512–10522. [CrossRef] [PubMed]

7. Fallowfield, J.A. Therapeutic targets in liver fibrosis. *Am. J. Physiol. Gastrointest. Liver Physiol.* **2011**, *300*, G709–G715. [CrossRef] [PubMed]

8. Molinski, T.F.; Dalisay, D.S.; Lievens, S.L.; Saludes, J.P. Drug development from marine natural products. *Nat. Rev. Drug Discov.* **2009**, *8*, 69–85. [CrossRef] [PubMed]

9. Fitton, J.H. Therapies from fucoidan; multifunctional marine polymers. *Mar. Drugs* **2011**, *9*, 1731–1760. [CrossRef] [PubMed]

10. Nair, D.G.; Weiskirchen, R.; Al-Musharafi, S.K. The use of marine-derived bioactive compounds as potential hepatoprotective agents. *Acta Pharmacol. Sin.* **2015**, *36*, 158–170. [CrossRef] [PubMed]

11. Chang, Y.C.; Kuo, L.M.; Hwang, T.L.; Yeh, J.; Wen, Z.H.; Fang, L.S.; Wu, Y.C.; Lin, C.S.; Sheu, J.H.; Sung, P.J. Pinnisterols A–C, New 9,11-Secosterols from a Gorgonian *Pinnigorgia* sp. *Mar. Drugs* **2016**, *14*, 12. [CrossRef] [PubMed]

12. Chang, H.H.; Chang, Y.C.; Chen, W.F.; Hwang, T.L.; Fang, L.S.; Wen, Z.H.; Chen, Y.H.; Wu, Y.C.; Sung, P.J. Pubinernoid A and Apo-9′-fucoxanthinone, Secondary Metabolites from a Gorgonian Coral *Pinnigorgia* sp. *Nat. Prod. Commun.* **2016**, *11*, 707–708. [PubMed]

13. Chang, Y.C.; Hwang, T.L.; Sheu, J.H.; Wu, Y.C.; Sung, P.J. New Anti-Inflammatory 9,11-Secosterols with a Rare Tricyclo [5,2,1,1] decane Ring from a Formosan Gorgonian *Pinnigorgia* sp. *Mar. Drugs* **2016**, *14*, 218. [CrossRef] [PubMed]

14. Chang, Y.C.; Hwang, T.L.; Chao, C.H.; Sung, P.J. New Marine Sterols from a Gorgonian *Pinnigorgia* sp. *Molecules* **2017**, *22*, 393. [CrossRef] [PubMed]

15. Chang, Y.C.; Hwang, T.L.; Kuo, L.M.; Sung, P.J. Pinnisterols D–J, New 11-Acetoxy-9,11-secosterols with a 1,4-Quinone Moiety from Formosan Gorgonian Coral *Pinnigorgia* sp. (Gorgoniidae). *Mar. Drugs* **2017**, *15*, 11. [CrossRef] [PubMed]

16. Chang, Y.; Kuo, L.; Su, J.; Hwang, T.; Kuo, Y.; Lin, C.; Wu, Y.; Sheu, J.; Sung, P. Pinnigorgiols A–C, 9,11-secosterols with a rare ring arrangement from a gorgonian coral *Pinnigorgia* sp. *Tetrahedron* **2016**, *72*, 999–1004. [CrossRef]

17. Brunati, A.M.; Pagano, M.A.; Bindoli, A.; Rigobello, M.P. Thiol redox systems and protein kinases in hepatic stellate cell regulatory processes. *Free Radic. Res.* **2010**, *44*, 363–378. [CrossRef] [PubMed]

18. Dunning, S.; Ur Rehman, A.; Tiebosch, M.H.; Hannivoort, R.A.; Haijer, F.W.; Woudenberg, J.; van den Heuvel, F.A.; Buist-Homan, M.; Faber, K.N.; Moshage, H. Glutathione and antioxidant enzymes serve complementary roles in protecting activated hepatic stellate cells against hydrogen peroxide-induced cell death. *Biochim. Biophys. Acta* **2013**, *1832*, 2027–2034. [CrossRef] [PubMed]

19. Circu, M.L.; Aw, T.Y. Glutathione and apoptosis. *Free Radic. Res.* **2008**, *42*, 689–706. [CrossRef] [PubMed]

20. Kuo, L.M.; Kuo, C.Y.; Lin, C.Y.; Hung, M.F.; Shen, J.J.; Hwang, T.L. Intracellular glutathione depletion by oridonin leads to apoptosis in hepatic stellate cells. *Molecules* **2014**, *19*, 3327–3344. [CrossRef] [PubMed]

21. Dong, H.; Guo, H.; Liang, Y.; Wang, X.; Niu, Y. Astragaloside IV synergizes with ferulic acid to suppress hepatic stellate cells activation in vitro. *Free Radic. Res.* **2017**, *51*, 167–178. [CrossRef] [PubMed]

22. Huang, Y.; Li, X.; Wang, Y.; Wang, H.; Huang, C.; Li, J. Endoplasmic reticulum stress-induced hepatic stellate cell apoptosis through calcium-mediated JNK/P38 MAPK and Calpain/Caspase-12 pathways. *Mol. Cell. Biochem.* **2014**, *394*, 1–12. [CrossRef] [PubMed]

23. Brenner, C.; Galluzzi, L.; Kepp, O.; Kroemer, G. Decoding cell death signals in liver inflammation. *J. Hepatol.* **2013**, *59*, 583–594. [CrossRef] [PubMed]

24. Takeda, K.; Naguro, I.; Nishitoh, H.; Matsuzawa, A.; Ichijo, H. Apoptosis signaling kinases: From stress response to health outcomes. *Antioxid. Redox Signal.* **2011**, *15*, 719–761. [CrossRef] [PubMed]

25. Sun, X.; Zhang, X.; Hu, H.; Lu, Y.; Chen, J.; Yasuda, K.; Wang, H. Berberine inhibits hepatic stellate cell proliferation and prevents experimental liver fibrosis. *Biol. Pharm. Bull.* **2009**, *32*, 1533–1537. [CrossRef] [PubMed]

26. Wasmuth, H.E.; Tacke, F.; Trautwein, C. Chemokines in liver inflammation and fibrosis. *Semin. Liver Dis.* **2010**, *30*, 215–225. [CrossRef] [PubMed]

27. Puche, J.E.; Saiman, Y.; Friedman, S.L. Hepatic stellate cells and liver fibrosis. *Compr. Physiol.* **2013**, *3*, 1473–1492. [PubMed]

28. Ray, K. Liver: Hepatic stellate cells hold the key to liver fibrosis. *Nat. Rev. Gastroenterol. Hepatol.* **2014**, *11*, 74. [CrossRef] [PubMed]

29. Kim, S.Y.; Kang, K.L.; Lee, J.C.; Heo, J.S. Nicotinic acetylcholine receptor alpha7 and beta4 subunits contribute nicotine-induced apoptosis in periodontal ligament stem cells. *Mol. Cells* **2012**, *33*, 343–350. [CrossRef] [PubMed]

30. Pamenter, M.E.; Perkins, G.A.; Gu, X.Q.; Ellisman, M.H.; Haddad, G.G. DIDS (4,4-diisothiocyanatostilbene disulphonic acid) induces apoptotic cell death in a hippocampal neuronal cell line and is not neuroprotective against ischemic stress. *PLoS ONE* **2013**, *8*, e60804. [CrossRef] [PubMed]

31. Posadas, I.; Santos, P.; Cena, V. Acetaminophen induces human neuroblastoma cell death through NFKB activation. *PLoS ONE* **2012**, *7*, e50160. [CrossRef] [PubMed]

32. Ricci, C.; Pastukh, V.; Leonard, J.; Turrens, J.; Wilson, G.; Schaffer, D.; Schaffer, S.W. Mitochondrial DNA damage triggers mitochondrial-superoxide generation and apoptosis. *Am. J. Physiol. Cell Physiol.* **2008**, *294*, C413–C422. [CrossRef] [PubMed]

33. Crosas-Molist, E.; Fabregat, I. Role of NADPH oxidases in the redox biology of liver fibrosis. *Redox Biol.* **2015**, *6*, 106–111. [CrossRef] [PubMed]

34. Wang, K. Autophagy and apoptosis in liver injury. *Cell Cycle* **2015**, *14*, 1631–1642. [CrossRef] [PubMed]

35. Siegmund, S.V.; Qian, T.; de Minicis, S.; Harvey-White, J.; Kunos, G.; Vinod, K.Y.; Hungund, B.; Schwabe, R.F. The endocannabinoid 2-arachidonoyl glycerol induces death of hepatic stellate cells via mitochondrial reactive oxygen species. *FASEB J.* **2007**, *21*, 2798–2806. [CrossRef] [PubMed]

36. Chowdhury, A.A.; Chaudhuri, J.; Biswas, N.; Manna, A.; Chatterjee, S.; Mahato, S.K.; Chaudhuri, U.; Jaisankar, P.; Bandyopadhyay, S. Synergistic apoptosis of CML cells by buthionine sulfoximine and hydroxychavicol correlates with activation of AIF and GSH-ROS-JNK-ERK-iNOS pathway. *PLoS ONE* **2013**, *8*, e73672. [CrossRef] [PubMed]

37. Huang, J.; Wu, L.; Tashiro, S.; Onodera, S.; Ikejima, T. Reactive oxygen species mediate oridonin-induced HepG2 apoptosis through p53, MAPK, and mitochondrial signaling pathways. *J. Pharmacol. Sci.* **2008**, *107*, 370–379. [CrossRef] [PubMed]

38. Szuster-Ciesielska, A.; Mizerska-Dudka, M.; Daniluk, J.; Kandefer-Szerszen, M. Butein inhibits ethanol-induced activation of liver stellate cells through TGF-beta, NFkappaB, p38, and JNK signaling pathways and inhibition of oxidative stress. *J. Gastroenterol.* **2013**, *48*, 222–237. [CrossRef] [PubMed]

39. Schnabl, B.; Bradham, C.A.; Bennett, B.L.; Manning, A.M.; Stefanovic, B.; Brenner, D.A. TAK1/JNK and p38 have opposite effects on rat hepatic stellate cells. *Hepatology* **2001**, *34*, 953–963. [CrossRef] [PubMed]

40. Jameel, N.M.; Thirunavukkarasu, C.; Wu, T.; Watkins, S.C.; Friedman, S.L.; Gandhi, C.R. p38-MAPK- and caspase-3-mediated superoxide-induced apoptosis of rat hepatic stellate cells: Reversal by retinoic acid. *J. Cell. Physiol.* **2009**, *218*, 157–166. [CrossRef] [PubMed]

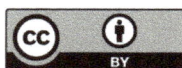

![marine drugs logo] *marine drugs*

MDPI

Article

The Protective Role of Sulfated Polysaccharides from Green Seaweed *Udotea flabellum* in Cells Exposed to Oxidative Damage

Fernando Bastos Presa [1,2,†], Maxsuell Lucas Mendes Marques [1,2,†], Rony Lucas Silva Viana [1], Leonardo Thiago Duarte Barreto Nobre [1], Leandro Silva Costa [3] and Hugo Alexandre Oliveira Rocha [1,2,*]

[1] Departamento de Bioquímica, Universidade Federal do Rio Grande do Norte, Natal 59078-970, Rio Grande do Norte, Brazil; fernandobpresa@gmail.com (F.B.P.); maxsuell_lucas@hotmail.com (M.L.M.M.); rony_lucas@hotmail.com (R.L.S.V.); leo.dnobre@gmail.com (L.T.D.B.N.)
[2] Programa de Pós-graduação em Ciências da Saúde, Universidade Federal do Rio Grande do Norte, Natal 59078-970, Rio Grande do Norte, Brazil
[3] Instituto Federal de Educação, Ciência, e Tecnologia do Rio Grande do Norte (IFRN), Ceara-Mirim 59900-000, Rio Grande do Norte, Brazil; leandro-silva-costa@hotmail.com
* Correspondence: hugo@cb.ufrn.br; Tel.: +55-84-3215-3416
† These authors contributed equally.

Received: 16 March 2018; Accepted: 14 April 2018; Published: 20 April 2018

Abstract: Seaweed is a rich source of bioactive sulfated polysaccharides. We obtained six sulfated polysaccharide-rich fractions (UF-0.3, UF-0.5, UF-0.6, UF-0.7, UF-1.0, and UF-2.0) from the green seaweed *Udotea flabellum* (UF) by proteolytic digestion followed by sequential acetone precipitation. Biochemical analysis of these fractions showed that they were enriched with sulfated galactans. The viability and proliferative capacity of 3T3 fibroblasts exposed to $FeSO_4$ (2 μM), $CuSO_4$ (1 μM) or ascorbate (2 mM) was not affected. However, these cells were exposed to oxidative stress in the presence of $FeSO_4$ or $CuSO_4$ and ascorbate, which caused the activation of caspase-3 and caspase-9, resulting in apoptosis of the cells. We also observed increased lipid peroxidation, evaluated by the detection of malondialdehyde and decreased glutathione and superoxide dismutase levels. Treating the cells with the ultrafiltrate fractions (UF) fractions protected the cells from the oxidative damage caused by the two salts and ascorbate. The most effective protection against the oxidative damage caused by iron was provided by UF-0.7 (1.0 mg/mL); on treatment with UF-0.7, cell viability was 55%. In the case of copper, cell viability on treatment with UF-0.7 was ~80%, but the most effective fraction in this model was UF-2.0, with cell viability of more than 90%. The fractions, mainly UF-0.7 and UF-2.0, showed low iron chelating activity, but high copper chelating activity and total antioxidant capacity (TAC). These results suggested that some of their protective mechanisms stem from these properties.

Keywords: sulfated galactan; 3T3 fibroblasts; green seaweed

---

1. Introduction

Copper and iron are two of the most abundant metals in the human body. They play several important roles in cellular metabolism. Copper is an essential micronutrient in human nutrition; it is a component of metalloenzymes and acts as an electron donor or acceptor, while iron forms complexes with proteins, such as flavin-iron enzymes, transferrin, ferritin, myoglobin or hemoglobin (responsible for oxygen transport), and with enzymes involved in electron transfer and oxidation-reduction reactions [1]. However, high levels of these transition metal ions in the form Cu^{2+} and Fe^{2+} are responsible for the production of reactive oxygen species (ROS), which leads to oxidative stress in cells, causing cellular damage and diseases. High levels of copper in the body, either by ingestion or genetic predisposition (Wilson's disease and Menkes syndrome), may contribute to mitochondrial dysfunction, subsequently leading to the production of ROS and induction of apoptosis. Consequently, several organs may suffer from its toxic effects [2]. An excess of iron in the body results in disorders, such as cirrhosis, liver cancer, diabetes, arrhythmia, and osteoporosis [3]. The use of chelating agents is always recommended in case of excess of physiological copper or iron [4]. However, these agents have several side effects [5]; thus, there is a continued search for new chelating agents.

Campo and colleagues [6] demonstrated that glycosaminoglycans, a group of sulfated polysaccharides (SPs), have antioxidant activity and can chelate both Cu^{++} and Fe^{++}, indicating that these compounds may serve as prospective drugs to combat the damaging effects of copper and iron. However, glycosaminoglycans are found in small amounts in all their sources, which could make their commercial use difficult. Other SPs are found in all seaweeds, and in some species of animals, plants, bacteria, fungi, and other microorganisms [7]. However, only seaweeds can synthetize SPs in large quantities. In addition, several SPs from seaweeds showed iron chelation activity, which makes seaweeds potential sources of chelating SPs.

Ulvans, green seaweed-origin SPs from the genus *Ulva*, showed antioxidant activity in several in vitro models [8]. In the present study, we draw attention to the SPs from *Ulva pertusa*, as they are known to form chelates with iron [9]. We have previously demonstrated that SPs from tropical green seaweeds, namely *Caulerpa cupressoides* [10], *Caulerpa prolifera* and *Caulerpa sertularioides* [11], have iron chelation activity.

Green seaweeds synthesize a range of sulfated homo- [12] and heteropolysaccharides [13]. These SPs have distinct chemistries and functions without parallelism in other organisms. This uniqueness results in the low degree of redundancy in the structure and mechanism of action of SPs, which has in turn resulted in renewed interest in the recognition of green seaweeds as novel sources of SPs [14]. However, there are fewer studies on SPs of green algae compared to those on other types of seaweed.

Recently, we found that an extract enriched in SPs from another tropical seaweed, *Udotea flabellum*, showed copper chelating activity (unpublished data). This seaweed is found easily on the Brazilian coast, and antioxidative properties of polysaccharides from its extracts have not been evaluated to date. Therefore, the aim of this study was to obtain SP-rich fractions from *U. flabellum* and evaluate their potential as protective agents in two models of oxidative stress caused by the presence of copper or iron.

2. Results

2.1. Chemical Analyses

We used a low-cost, widely reproducible method, which combined proteolysis and sequential acetone precipitation, to obtain six sulfated polysaccharide-rich fractions (named UF-0.3, UF-0.5, UF-0.6, UF-0.7, UF-1.0, and UF-2.0) from the green seaweed *U. flabellum*. The results of the chemical analysis of the fractions and their polysaccharide yields are summarized in Table 1. The yield ranged from 4.2% (UF-0.3) to 36.9% (UF-0.5); UF-0.3 and UF-1.0 were contaminated with proteins. The sulfate percentage indicated that it was present in all fractions.

Table 1. Chemical composition of polysaccharides extracted from the *U. flabellum*; Gal: galactose; Xyl: xylose; Man: mannose; Gluc: glucose; -Traces; n.d—not detected.

Sulfated Polysaccharides	Yield [a] (%)	Sulfate (%)	Protein (%)	Molar Ratio			
				Gal	Glu	Man	Xyl
UF-0.3	4.20	7.3 ± 0.8	4.9 ± 0.8	1.0	1.1	n.d	n.d
UF-0.5	36.9	18.7 ± 0.8	-	1.0	0.5	-	-
UF-0.6	9.9	10.7 ± 1.2	n.d	1.0	0.4	0.2	-
UF-0.7	17.7	17.0 ± 1.8	-	1.0	0.4	0.2	-
UF-1.0	11.5	9.8 ± 0.7	5.6 ± 0.8	1.0	0.7	0.7	0.3
UF-2.0	19.7	21.5 ± 1.3	n.d	1.0	1.0	1.0	n.d

[a] All polysaccharides obtained by acetone precipitation were dried and weighed and total mass of each sample corresponded to 100%.

In order to confirm whether the sulfate was covalently linked to polysaccharides, we subjected the fractions to agarose gel electrophoresis. After the gel was stained with toluidine blue (Figure 1) we found that all fractions contained electrophoretically mobile purple colored bands, characteristic to sulfated polysaccharides. We observed slight differences in the mobility of the bands of each fraction, and multiple bands were observed for some fractions (UF-0.3 and UF-1.0).

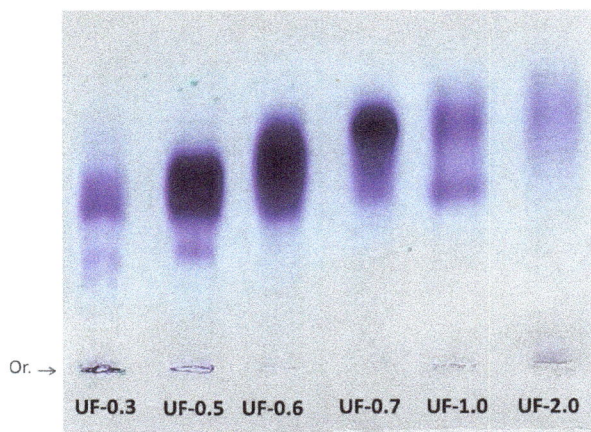

Figure 1. Electrophoresis in 0.05 M diaminopropane acetate buffer, pH 9.0, of fractions obtained by acetone precipitation. About 5 μL (50 μg) of each polysaccharide was applied in agarose gel prepared in diaminopropane acetate buffer and subjected to electrophoresis, as described in methods. Or.—origin.

Table 1 also shows that galactose and glucose are present in all fractions, but in different proportions. Galactose was found to be the predominant sugar in all fractions; therefore, it was chosen as a reference to determine the proportion of other sugars. Glucose was found in large proportions in the fractions UF-0.3, UF-1.0, and UF-2.0. Mannose was not detected in UF-0.3, and its percentage increased with respect to other sugars in subsequent fractions reaching the maximum in UF-2.0. Xylose was absent in fractions UF-0.3 and UF-2.0.

2.2. Effect of Sulfated Polisaccharides on Cell Viability and Cell Proliferation

Initially, we evaluated whether sulfated polysaccharides were toxic to 3T3 fibroblast cells. As seen in Figure 2A, the polysaccharides, at the proportions determined previously, failed to have any effect on the ability of fibroblasts to reduce 3-(4,5-dimethylthiazol-2-yl)-2,5-diphenyltetrazolium bromide

(MTT). In contrast, treatment with cisplatin, which was used as a positive control, caused 3T3 cells to reduce only 27% of the MTT molecules.

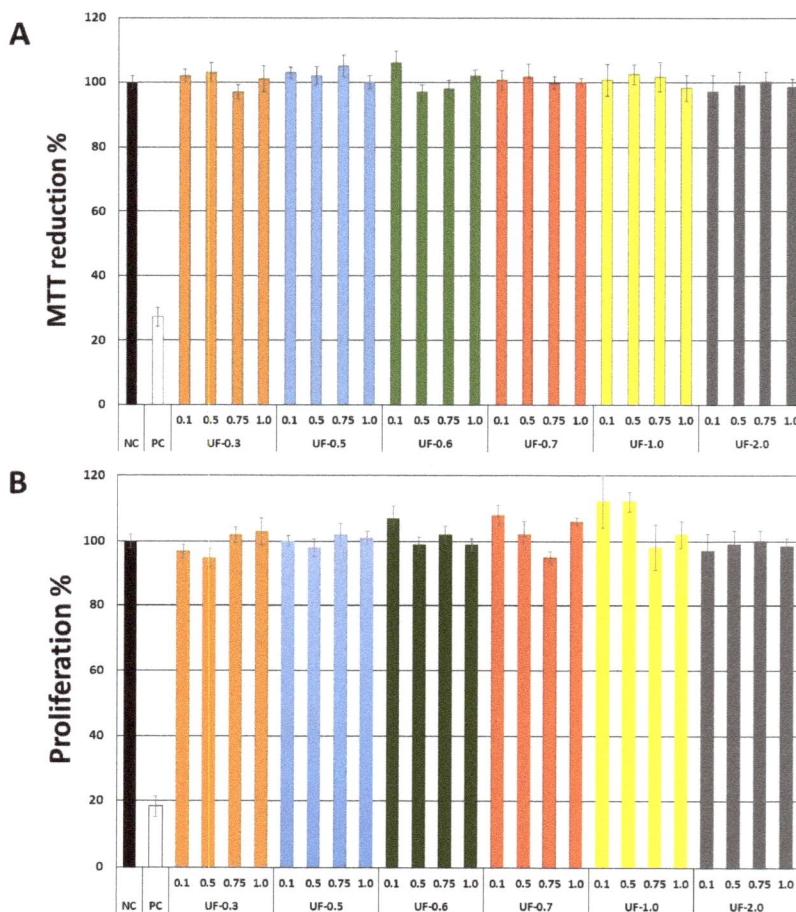

Figure 2. Effect of different concentrations (mg/mL) of sulfated polysaccharides from *U. flabellum* on the ability of fibroblast (3T3) cells to reduce 3-(4,5-dimethylthiazol-2-yl)-2,5-diphenyltetrazolium bromide (MTT) (**A**) and incorporate 5-bromo-2-deoxyuridine (BrdU) BrdU (**B**). NC—negative control composed only of culture medium with fetal bovine serum. PC—positive control-culture medium with fetal bovine serum and cisplatin (2 μg/mL).

Figure 2B shows that the sulfated polysaccharides also did not affect the proliferation of 3T3 cells, as the incorporation of 5-bromo-2-deoxyuridine (BrdU) by the cells incubated in the presence of fractions was similar with the cells of the negative control group (cells exposed only to medium and fetal bovine serum).

2.3. Evaluation of SP Chelation Activity

As UF-0.3 and UF-1.0 showed protein contamination, we did not use these fractions in subsequent experiments.

As seen in Figure 3, all samples had low iron chelating activity (<20%) compared to that of ethylenediaminetetraacetic acid (EDTA), used as the positive control. In contrast, the polysaccharides showed a dose-dependent effect when copper was used. The most significant chelation (~90%) was observed for UF-2.0.

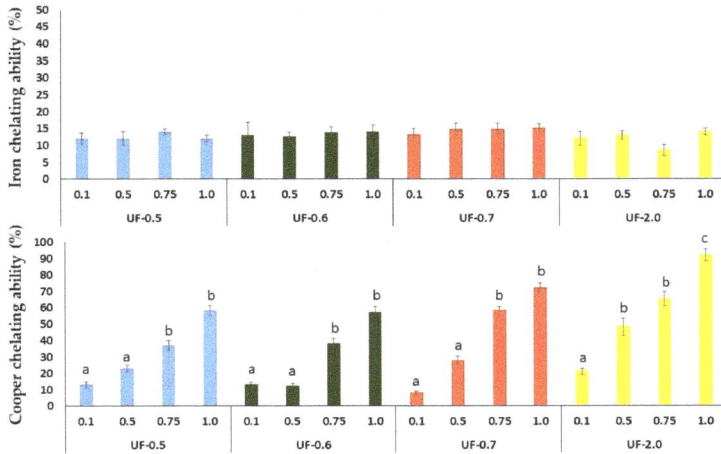

Figure 3. Copper- and iron-chelating ability of sulfated polysaccharides from *U. flabellum*. Data are presented as means ± standard deviation. Different lowercase letters indicate a significant difference ($p < 0.05$) between the ability of polysaccharides to chelate copper or iron. Ethylenediaminetetraacetic acid (EDTA) was used as the positive control, which corresponded to 100% chelating ability (maximum chelating ability was 0.025 and 0.02 mg/mL in the copper and iron analyses, respectively).

2.4. Effect of Sulfated Polysaccharides on MTT Reduction in 3T3 Fibroblast Cells

As Figure 4 shows, the sulfated polysaccharides protected the cells from the action of $FeSO_4$ and $CuSO_4$ -. On using $FeSO_4$, UF-0.7 was the only fraction that caused the 3T3 cells to reduce more than 50% of the MTT molecules that were present in the culture medium. In contrast, when we used $CuSO_4$, the cells that were subjected to the higher concentrations of samples were able to reduce more than 50% of the MTT molecules. Notably, fractions UF-0.7 and UF-2.0, (1.0 mg/mL) enabled cells to reduce ~81% and ~95% of the MTT molecules, respectively.

We also exposed the 3T3 cells to $FeSO_4$ (2 µM), $CuSO_4$ (1 µM) or ascorbate (2 mM) and we observed that the ability of 3T3 cells to reduce MTT was not affected in any of the conditions evaluated.

2.5. Effect of Sulfated Polysaccharides on 3T3 Fibroblast Caspase-3 and Caspase-9

Several studies show that $FeSO_4$ and $CuSO_4$ induce cell death along with ascorbate by promoting the activation of caspases. Therefore, we evaluated the activity of capase-3 and caspase-9 from the 3T3 fibroblasts that were exposed to $FeSO_4$ and $CuSO_4$, in the absence and presence of sulfated polysaccharides (1 mg/mL). Figure 5 shows that the activity of caspase-3 and caspase-9 is very high after the cells have been exposed to oxidizing conditions positive control (PC), metal plus ascorbate). Moreover, the presence of polysaccharides decreased the activity of both caspases in various conditions. However, polysaccharides were less effective when the cells were exposed to $FeSO_4$ than when exposed to $CuSO_4$.

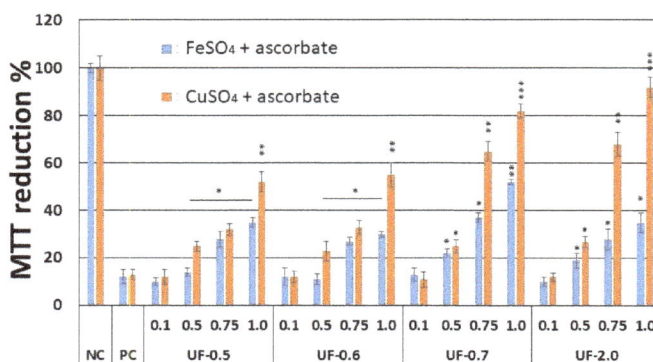

Figure 4. Effect of different amounts (mg/mL) of sulfated polysaccharides from *U. flabellum* on the ability of fibroblast (3T3) cells to reduce MTT in the two models of oxidative stress. NC—negative control composed only of culture medium with fetal bovine serum. PC—positive control-culture medium with fetal bovine serum, FeSO$_4$ or CuSO$_4$, and ascorbate. *** $p < 0.001$; ** $p < 0.01$; * $p < 0.05$ vs. PC.

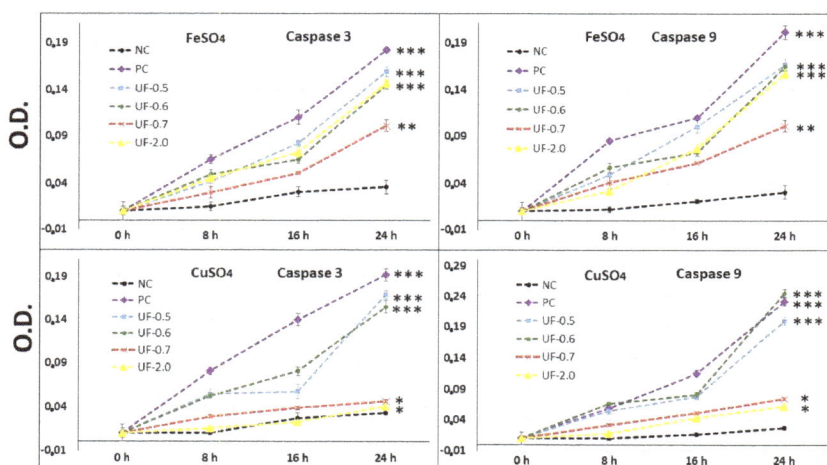

Figure 5. Effect of different amounts (mg/mL) of sulfated polysaccharides from *U. flabellum* on caspase-3 and caspase-9 activity in 3T3 cells exposed to two models of oxidative stress. O.D.—optical density. NC—negative control composed only of culture medium with fetal bovine serum. PC—positive control-culture medium with fetal bovine serum FeSO$_4$ or CuSO$_4$ and ascorbate. *** $p < 0.001$; ** $p < 0.01$; * $p < 0.05$ vs. NC.

When the effect of each fraction was studied individually, the activity of the caspases in fractions UF-0.5, UF-0.6, and UF-2.0 in the presence of FeSO$_4$ was about 25% lower than that observed with the PC group. On the other hand, the activity of both caspases corresponded to about 50% to that observed in the PC group.

2.6. Lipid Peroxidation Analysis

Estimation of malondialdehyde levels was performed to determine the degree of free radical production in 3T3 cells (Table 2). The concentration of malondialdehyde found in the cells of the control group was approximately 250 mmol/10^6 cells, and this was considered to be the physiological concentration. These levels were about ten times higher in the presence of metals and ascorbate. This indicates that the presence of these compounds promoted oxidative damage.

Table 2. Evaluation of the protective effect of the polysaccharides on the 3T3 cells exposed to the two models of oxidative damage.

	Effect of Sulfated Polysaccharides (1 mg/mL) on Total Glutathione (GSH) (mmol/10^6 Cell) Levels of 3T3 Cells Exposed to Oxidative Damage		
		$FeSO_4$	$CuSO_4$
NC	6.78 ± 2.21		7.01 ± 2.11
PC		2.37 ± 0.60 [a]	2.47 ± 0.43 [a]
UF-0.5		3.63 ± 0.61 [b]	4.71 ± 1.01 [c]
UF-0.6		4.18 ± 0.98 [c]	4.52 ± 0.93 [c]
UF-0.7		4.75 ± 0.78 [c]	4.89 ± 1.12 [c]
UF-2.0		4.76 ± 1.08 [c]	5.77 ± 1.08 [c]
	Effect of Sulfated Polysaccharides (1 mg/mL) on Malondialdehyde (MDA) (mmol/10^6 cell) Levels of 3T3 Cells Exposed to Oxidative Damage		
		$FeSO_4$	$CuSO_4$
NC	250.1 ± 21.1		217.2 ± 41.7
PC		2123.8 ± 99.7 [a]	2312.1 ± 103.5 [a]
UF-0.5		1542.5 ± 123.1 [b]	1428.5 ± 111.2 [b]
UF-0.6		1488.1 ± 209.2 [b]	$15,012 \pm 93.9$ [b]
UF-0.7		1107.0 ± 89.1 [c]	1001 ± 101.1 [c]
UF-2.0		1083.0 ± 56.3 [c]	987 ± 95.1 [c]
	Effect of Sulfated Polysaccharides (1 mg/mL) on Total Superoxide Dismutase (SOD) Levels (U/mg Protein) of 3T3 Cells Exposed to Oxidative Damage		
		$FeSO_4$	$CuSO_4$
NC	33.5 ± 1.1		31.2 ± 0.9 [a]
PC		8.2 ± 2.1 [a]	10.2 ± 1.1 [a]
UF-0.5		11.8 ± 2.1 [b]	13.9 ± 1.5 [b]
UF-0.6		10.9 ± 1.0 [b]	14.7 ± 1.2 [b]
UF-0.7		14.2 ± 0.4 [b]	20.8 ± 1.5 [c]
UF-2.0		15.8 ± 0.7 [b]	20.9 ± 0.8 [c]

PC—positive control-culture medium with fetal bovine serum $FeSO_4$ or $CuSO_4$ and ascorbate. [a] $p < 0.001$ vs. NC; [b] $p < 0.05$; [c] $p < 0.001$ vs. PC.

When the cells were exposed to $FeSO_4$ or $CuSO_4$ and ascorbate along with the polysaccharides the levels of malondialdehyde were significantly lower than those observed in the PC group. The most efficient samples to reduce malondialdehyde levels were UF-0.7 and UF-2.0.

2.7. Assessment of the Cell Antioxidant Status

The concentration of glutathione (GSH) and Superoxide dismutase (SOD) were assayed in order to evaluate antioxidant balance after free radical production (Table 2). The levels of GSH (6.78 ± 2.21 mmol/10^6 cell) and SOD (33.5 ± 1.1 mmol/10^6 cell) found in the control cells were considered physiological. A significant reduction in levels of both antioxidants was observed in several experimental conditions, and this effect was more pronounced in the PC group.

When cells were treated with copper, ascorbate, and polysaccharides, we found no significant difference in GSH levels between the treated groups and the negative group (NC) group. When cells were exposed to iron, similar results were obtained with UF-0.7 and UF-2.0. This shows that these two fractions prevented a decrease in the levels of GSH even when the cells were subjected to oxidative damage.

The protective effect of polysaccharides was less pronounced in the case of SOD. However, treatment with both UF-0.7 and UF-2.0, in the presence of iron or copper, showed decreased levels of this enzyme

2.8. In Vitro Evaluation of Antioxidant Capacity of Polysaccharides

The total antioxidant capacity (TAC) test aims to evaluate the ability of a compound to donate electrons to another molecule, which stabilizes it. UF-2.0 presented significantly lower TAC than the other samples. The other samples presented significantly similar TAC as shown in Figure 6.

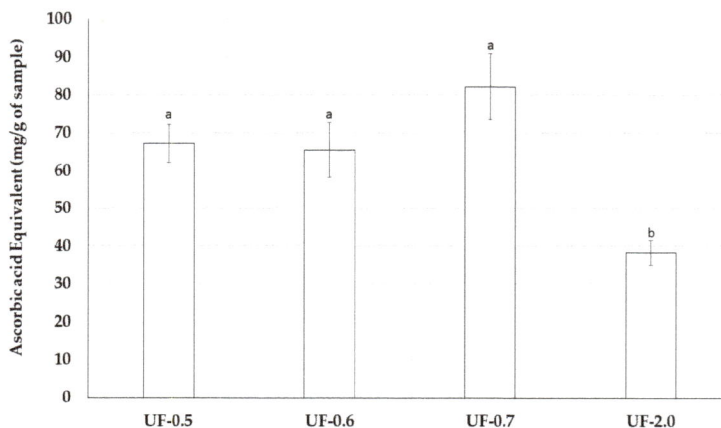

Figure 6. Total antioxidant capacity of sulfated polysaccharides-rich fractions from *U. flabellum.* Data are presented as means ± standard deviation. [a,b] Different lowercase letters indicate a significant difference ($p < 0.05$) between the total antioxidant capacities of samples.

The polysaccharides at all concentrations tested (from 0.1 to 1.0 mg/mL) did not exhibit any hydroxyl radical scavenging activity. In addition, only UF-2.0 exhibited superoxide radical scavenging activity, but this activity was 15%, and it was only detected at the highest concentration (1.0 mg/mL).

The last antioxidant evaluation test we performed was to determine the reducing power of the samples. UF-0.5 and UF-2.0 showed activity (~35%), but we only detected this activity at the highest concentration (1.0 mg/mL).

3. Discussion

The data presented in Table 1 indicate that all fractions contained polysaccharides and sulfate. The confirmation that sulfate ions were covalently bound to the polysaccharides was achieved by using agarose gel electrophoresis, as the free sulfate ions and small sulfated molecules would not be retained in the gel mesh [15]. Based on these data, we obtained six sulfated polysaccharide-rich fractions from *U. flabellum*.

We obtained the fractions using differential precipitation with acetone, which was due to different interaction forces between polysaccharide molecules with water. Therefore, the addition of increasing volumes of acetone to the samples is necessary during precipitation. The polysaccharides, which are most weakly bound, precipitate with lower concentrations of acetone and those, which are more strongly bound, requiring higher concentrations of acetone for precipitation.

Agarose gel electrophoresis allowed the visualization and verification of the existence of sulfated polysaccharides in all fractions. The purple color obtained is typical of SPs due to the interaction of the toluidine blue dye with the sulfated group present in the polysaccharides [15].

Generally, in agarose gel electrophoresis systems, the mobility of the polysaccharides depends on their charges; for example, the more negative ones have greater mobility than the negative ones. However, as suggested by Dietrich and Dietrich [15], the use of 1,3-diaminopropane was important for the visualization of different polysaccharide molecules in the fractions. In the pH of the test (9.0) the sulfated polysaccharides assume a conformation in which some sulfate groups are exposed and others not. These exposed sulfates react with the diamine and their negative charges are quenched. This will induce a change in the conformation of the polysaccharide, and new sulfate groups are exposed and, accordingly, will react with the diamine. This process continues until equilibrium is reached, and the conformation of the polysaccharide no longer changes. However, the polysaccharide, in this conformational equilibrium condition, will still have sulfate groups that did not react with the diamine, and it will be these groups that will permit the mobility of the polysaccharide in the agarose during the electrophoresis. In short, polysaccharide molecules that have the same structure will have the same interaction with the diamine, and consequently have the same electrophoretic motility; whereas, structurally different polysaccharides have different electrophoretic mobilities [15]. In Figure 2, the presence of multiple bands with different mobilities in some fractions indicated that there are at least two polysaccharides in these Udotea fractions.

The results discussed so far (acetone precipitation, electrophoresis, and monosaccharide composition) show that *U. flabellum* synthesizes more than one type of sulfated polysaccharide. This agrees with reports that describe green seaweeds synthesizing more than one type of SP [13].

The analysis of the monosaccharide composition showed that all the fractions are heterogeneous, and that their main constituent is galactose. The predominance of one or more monomers over others as observed in the fractions of the *U. flabellum* was not surprising, as there are previous reports with data from other seaweeds, supporting a similar predominance [16,17]. Moreover, galactose has been described as the main component of SPs in other seaweeds, such as *Caulerpa cupressoides* [10] and *Codium isthmocladum* [12].

Our first objective was to rule out the toxicity of *Udotea* SPs to fibroblast 3T3 cells. As seen in Figure 2, *Udotea* SPs were not cytotoxic, and did not influence the proliferation of fibroblasts. Therefore, we hypothesized these SPs to be putative protective agents under conditions of oxidative stress. Two samples (UF-0.3 and UF-1.0) were not used due to protein contamination.

Production of reactive oxygen species leads to oxidative stress in cells, and, consequently, are harmful to organisms. In many oxidative stress models, one of the first reactive species of oxygen that is formed in great quantity is the superoxide anion. It is considered a reactive primary species, as it can generate reactive derivatives by direct interactions with other molecules or by processes catalyzed by metals or enzymes. In addition, under conditions of stress, superoxide anions can interact with proteins with iron as a cofactor and release iron groups from them [18]. Superoxide anion is a substrate for SOD that transforms it into hydrogen peroxide. These two species have a short-lived action. However, they can react with iron or copper through the Fenton and Haber-Weiss reactions, which leads to formation of the hydroxyl radical (OH•), which is a much more damaging ROS [19].

Several studies have demonstrated that the presence of iron or copper sulfate under culture conditions promotes oxidative stress. In addition, the presence of ascorbate also contributes to enhance the production of the detrimental OH• [6,20]. Therefore, we chose the model of cellular damage in the presence of these two salts and ascorbate to evaluate the protective action of Udotea SPs.

Because the oxidation of a substrate is caused by a reactive species in a chain reaction that includes three steps (initiation, propagation, and termination), the action of the antioxidants is evaluated through several mechanisms. Chelating agents act in both the initiation and propagation steps. Thus, they are antioxidant compounds because they prevent the formation of radicals and thus indirectly reduce the risk posed by radicals [9].

That is why we evaluated the chelating capacity of *Udotea* SPs. All SPs showed high copper chelating activity, with emphasis on UF-0.7 and UF-2.0 at 1 mg/mL, which presented activities superior to 80% and 90%, respectively. SPs from the brown seaweed *Undaria pinnatifida* also showed high copper chelating activity, but this activity was obtained only with high concentration (2.5 mg/mL) [21]. SPs from *Dictyopteris justii* (brown seaweed) also showed iron chelating activity, and one of these polysaccharides had a maximum activity of ~80% (1 mg/mL) [22]. We have not identified other reports that have evaluated the copper chelating activity of SPs from seaweeds. Many reports show a positive correlation between the activity of SPs and their sulfate content. We did not identify this correlation with *Udotea* SPs. Indeed, the copper chelating activity of polysaccharides appears to be more related to the conformation of the polysaccharide than to the presence of negatively charged groups, since neutral polysaccharides showed this activity. For example, yeast-neutral polysaccharides showed 80% activity when evaluated at concentrations similar to those used in the present study [23].

This copper chelating activity of *Udotea* SPS was reflected in cell-based assays. We found that UF-0.7 and UF-2.0, which were the most potent chelators, were also the ones that most protected the cells from damage caused by oxidative stress. Moreover, as shown in Figure 3, this activity was dose dependent. UF-1.0 contained the most potent SPs, which was demonstrated when SPs were used at similar concentrations (Figures 4 and 5, and Table 2).

Campo and colleagues [6] showed that the glycosaminoglycans, hyaluronic acid and chondroitin-4-sulfate, protect fibroblastic cells against the damage caused by the presence of $CuSO_4$ and ascorbate. However, when we performed the cytotoxicity assay (Figure 4.), the rate of reduction of MTT was 80%, and this was only achieved at a concentration of 2.0 mg/mL, which is twice the concentration used with UF-2.0. In addition, with UF-2.0, we achieved an MTT reduction rate of over 90%.

Our results showed that when 3T3 cells were exposed to $CuSO_4$, the levels of caspase-3 (executioner) and caspase-9 (initiator) in the cells were very high, corroborating with the MTT test data (Figure 5). This implies that the cells under conditions of oxidative damage tend to die by apoptosis. Caspases are a group of proteases important for cellular apoptosis to occur. There are initiator caspases and executioner caspases, which are activated by the initiator caspases. The activation of caspases under conditions of oxidative stress and their involvement in the process of cell death induced by it have been reported since a long time [24]. The activity levels of these caspases in the groups of cells treated with UF-0.7 and UF-2.0 were similar to those observed in the NC group. This data demonstrated that fractions UF-0.7 and UF-2.0 could act as chelating agents, thus decreasing the oxidative stress, activation of caspases, and the number of dead cells (as seen indirectly via the MTT test).

To confirm that the oxidative stress in the cells was reduced by the presence of sulfated polysaccharides, we evaluated the levels of three markers of oxidative stress SOD, GSH, and malondialdehyde.

Free radical-mediated cell damage can generally cause lipid peroxidation, and malondialdehyde levels are a good marker of this event, the higher the amount of this molecule, the greater the lipid peroxidation [6]. The presence of sulfated polysaccharides prevented the levels of malondialdehyde from getting so high. In fractions UF-0.7 and UF-2.0, these levels were only 5 times higher than those observed in the PC.

The concentration of SOD and GSH decreases considerably when cells are exposed to oxidative damage. This is because SOD and GSH are consumed by the reactive species that are formed [25].

This explains the decrease in the levels of SOD and GSH when 3T3 cells are exposed to oxidative damage. In both cases, we observed that the sulfated polysaccharides, mainly UF-0.7 and UF-2.0, protected the cells against the oxidative damage.

The mechanism by which SPs from *Udotea* reduce cellular damage against free radical overproduction is similar to that of hyaluronic acid and chondroitin-4-sulfate, typical SPs that can behave as chelating agents [6,26]. We had hypothesized that the protective action of polysaccharides from this seaweed against oxidative damage occurs mainly because of its copper chelating properties.

Udotea SPs presented low iron chelating activity. However, their presence protected 3T3 cells against oxidative damage caused by exposure to $FeSO_4$. This was observed in all the tests performed. In addition, the data showed that, unlike in the $CuSO_4$ assays, the most effective polysaccharide was UF-0.7. These data indicated that oxidative stress caused by iron was attenuated by the polysaccharides via other mechanisms besides chelation to wield their antioxidant action, consequently, protecting the cell against oxidative damage.

Therefore, we assessed antioxidant properties of *Udotea* SPs using five antioxidant tests. *Udotea* SPs were effective only in the TAC. In this test, we verified that the activity of UF-2.0 was lower than that of the other SPs. In contrast, UF-0.7 was the most potent antioxidant among all SPs. In the TAC assay, the sample is evaluated as an electron donor; the higher the value obtained in the TAC, the greater its ability to donate electrons and, consequently, to neutralize the ROS.

TAC data may partly explain why *Udotea* SPs, although not strong iron chelators, are able to protect cells from the oxidative stress caused by the presence of iron. We are interested in identifying other mechanisms that allow the *Udotea* SPs to act as protectors of cells exposed to oxidative stress caused by iron.

4. Materials and Methods

4.1. Materials

Iron (II) sulfate, potassium ferricianyde, sulfuric acid and acetonitrile were obtained from Merck (Darmstadt, Germany). Nitro Blue Tetrazolium (NBT), monosaccharides, methionine and ammonium molybdate were purchased from Sigma-Aldrich Co. (St. Louis, MO, USA). Cell culture medium components (Dulbecco's Modified Eagle Medium-DMEM), trypsin and newborn calf serum (FCS) were obtained from Cultilab (Campinas, Brazil). L-glutamine, sodium bicarbonate, sodium pyruvate and phosphate buffered saline (PBS) were purchased from Invitrogen Corporation (Burlington, ON, USA). All other solvents and chemicals were of analytical grade.

Eukaryotic cells—Mouse embryonic fibroblast cells (NIH/3T3 ATCC® CRL-1658™-3T3, Manassas, VA, USA) were grown in Dulbecco's modified Eagle's medium (DMEM) with 10% of fetal bovine serum (FBS), 10 mg/mL streptomycin, and 10,000 IU penicillin.

4.2. Extraction of Sulfated Polysaccharide-Rich Fractions

The seaweed *Udotea flabellum* was collected at Búzios Beach, Nísia Floresta-RN, Brazil. The alga was stored in our laboratory and dried at 50 °C under ventilation in an oven, ground in a blender and incubated with ethanol to eliminate lipids and pigments. About 90 g of powdered alga was suspended with five volumes of 0.25 M NaCl and the pH was adjusted to 8.0 with NaOH. Next, 900 mg of Prolav 750 (Prozyn Biosolutions, São Paulo, SP, Brazil), a mixture of alkaline proteases, was added for proteolytic digestion. After incubation for 24 h at 60 °C under agitation and periodical pH adjustments, the mixture was filtered through cheesecloth. The filtrate was fractionated by precipitation with acetone as follows: 0.3 volumes of ice-cold acetone was added to the solution under gentle agitation and maintained at 4 °C for 24 h. The precipitate formed was collected by centrifugation (10,000× *g*, 20 min), vacuum dried, resuspended in distilled water, and analyzed. The operation was repeated by adding 0.5, 0.6, 0.7, 1.0, and 2.0 volumes of acetone to the supernatant.

4.3. Chemical Analysis and Monosaccharide Composition

Sulfate content was determined according to the gelatin-barium method [27], using sodium sulfate (1 mg/mL) as standard and after acid hydrolysis of the polysaccharides (4 M HCl, 100 °C, 6 h). Protein content was measured using Spector's method [28]. The polysaccharides were hydrolyzed with 0.5, 1, 2, and 4 M, respectively, for various lengths of time, (0.5, 1, 2 and 4 h), at 100 °C. Reducing sugars were determined using the Somogyi-Nelson method [29]. After acid hydrolysis, sugar composition was determined by a LaChrom Elite® HPLC system from VWR-Hitachi (Hitachi, Ltd., Tokyo, Japan) with a refractive index detector (RI detector model L-2490). A LichroCART® 250-4 column (250 mm × 40 mm) packed with Lichrospher® 100 NH2 (5 μm) was coupled to the system. The sample mass used was 0.2 mg and analysis time was 25 min. The following sugars were analyzed as references: arabinose, fructose, fucose, galactose, glucose, glucosamine, glucuronic acid, mannose, and xylose.

4.4. 3-(4,5-dimethylthiazol-2-yl)-2,5-diphenyltetrazolium Bromide Test

For the tests, 0.5×10^4 cells were grown in 96-well plates with DMEM medium containing the samples in concentrations of 0.1, 0.5, 0.75 and 1 mg/mL for 24 h (each concentration in triplicate). The cell capacity to reduce MTT was determined by the colorimetric test of MTT as described earlier [30].

4.5. 5-bromo-2-deoxyuridine Incorporation

The cells (5×10^3 cells/well) were seeded into 96-well plates with 300 μL of fresh medium and incubated for 12 h at 37 °C and 5.0% CO_2. The medium was removed, the samples in DMEM medium was added to a final concentration between 0.1 and 1.0 mg/mL, and plates were incubated for 24 h, at 37 °C and 5.0% CO_2. After incubation, unbound samples were removed by washing the cells twice with 200 μL PBS and BrdU incorporation was determined according to manufacturer's instruction (BrdU cell proliferation assay kit-Cell Signaling, Danvers, MA, USA).

4.6. Induced Oxidative Stress Assay

3T3 cells (1×10^6 cells/mL) were placed in 6-well plates in de presence of 1 mL of DMEM supplemented with 10% FCS. After 24 h, the plates were washed and 1 mL of DMEM supplemented with 10% FCS and sulfated polysaccharides (0.1; 0.5; 0.75 or 1.0 mg/mL), $CuSO_4$ (1 μM, final concentration) or $FeSO_4$ (2 μM, final concentration) were added. 15 min after, 10 μL of 200 mM ascorbate acid (2 mM final concentration) was added. The plates were kept in culture condition (37 °C; 5% CO_2; dark) for 90 min; thus, the medium was replaced by 1 mL of the same fresh medium. After 24 h, the cells were submitted to MTT test as described above.

4.7. Caspase-3 and -9 Activity Assays

3T3 cells (1×10^6 cells/mL) were placed in 6-well plates in de presence of 1 mL of DMEM supplemented with 10% FCS. After 24 h, the plates were washed and 1 mL of DMEM supplemented with 10% FCS, $FeSO_4$, $CuSO_4$, ascorbate and/or sulfated polysaccharides (1 mg/mL) was added. After 90 min, the medium was replaced by fresh medium. 8, 16 and 24 h the plates were washed with ice-cold PBS and scraped into 200 mL lysis buffer (50 mM Tris-HCl (pH 7.4), 1% Tween 20, 0.25% sodium deoxycholate, 150 mM NaCl, 1 mM EDTA, 1 mM Na3VO4, 1 mM NaF], and protease inhibitors (1 mg/mL aprotinin, 10 mg/mL leupeptin and 1 mM 4-(2-aminoethyl) benzenesulfonyl fluoride) for 2 h in ice. The same conditions were used for untreated cells in the 0, 8, 16 and 24 h. Protein extracts were cleared by centrifugation and protein concentrations were determined using Bradford reagent [28] with bovine serum albumin as standard. In vitro caspase-3 and -9 protease activity was measured using a caspase activation kit according to the manufacturer's protocol (Invitrogen, São Paulo, Brazil). For this, 50 μL of cell lysate was mixed with 50 μL of 2x reaction buffer (containing 10 μL of 1 M dithiothreitol and 5 μL of 4 mM synthetic tetrapeptide Asp-Glue-Val (for caspase 3) or Leu-Glu-His-Asp (for caspase 9) conjugated top-nitroanilide (pNA)) in a 96-well plate, after which the mixture was incubated for 2 h at 37 °C in the dark. Active caspase cleaves the peptide and releases the chromophore pNA that can be detected spectrophotometrically at a wavelength of 405 nm. Theoretically, the apoptotic cell lysates containing active tested caspases should yield a considerable emission compared with the non-apoptotic cell lysates. Data presented are representative of those obtained in at least three independent experiments done in duplicates.

4.8. Superoxide Dismutase Evaluation

The SOD activity was measured using commercially available kit (SOD activity Enzo Life Sciences, Farmingdale, NY, USA). The principle of the method is based on the ability of SOD to neutralize superoxide ions created by the xanthine/xanthine oxidase system and subsequently inhibits the reduction of WST-1 (water soluble tetrazolium salt) to WST-1 formazan. Briefly, 3T3 fibroblasts (5×10^6 in six-well plate), obtained 24 h after oxidative stress induction, were washed with ice-cold

1× PBS, and lysed as described in kit protocol. The supernatant of each sample was collected, and the total SOD activity was assayed spectrophotometrically at 450 nm. SOD concentration, expressed in units per milligram of protein, was determined using the SOD standard curve.

4.9. Glutathione Evaluation

To assess the total level of glutathione, the 3T3 cells (5×10^6 in six-well plate), obtained 24 h after oxidative stress induction, were washed with ice-cold 1× PBS, removed, resuspended in PBS and centrifuged ($3000 \times g$ at 4 °C) twice for 5 min. After this process, the suspension obtained was then diluted in 50% trichloroacetic acid (Vetec, São Paulo, SP, Brazil) and centrifuged during 15 min ($3000 \times g$ at 4 °C). After, the cell supernatant was diluted with the same volume 0.4 M Tris buffer contained 0.01 M dithiobisnitrobenzoic (Sigma-Aldrich, São Paulo, SP, Brazil). The material was read at 412 nm. The results were expressed as nmol/10^6 cells.

4.10. Malonaldehyde Levels

To assess lipid peroxidation, malonaldehyde (MDA) production was measured with thiobarbituric acid reaction. Briefly, the cells under the same conditions as described above were triturated in 20 mM Tris-HCl buffer and centrifuged during 15 min ($3000 \times g$ at 4 °C). The chromogenic reagent (10.3 mM 1-methyl-2-phenylindole in acetonitrile, 3:1 *v/v*), and a 37% solution of HCl were dropped to each supernatant sample (150 mL). The samples were kept at 45 °C for 40 min, and then were centrifuged (15 min; $3000 \times g$; 4 °C). The absorbance was measured at 586 nm, and the results were expressed as nmol/10^6 cells.

4.11. Antioxidant Activity

Four assays were performed to analyze the antioxidant activity of the sulfated polysaccharides obtained: total antioxidant capacity, hydroxyl radical scavenging, superoxide radical scavenging, and ferric chelating, as previously described [11,23].

4.11.1. Determination of Total Antioxidant Capacity

This assay is based on the reduction of Mo (VI) to Mo (V) by sulfated polysaccharides and subsequent formation of a green phosphate/Mo(V) complex at acid pH. Tubes containing sulfated polysaccharides and reagent solution (0.6 M sulfuric acid, 28 mM sodium phosphate and 4 mM ammonium molybdate) were incubated at 95 °C for 90 min. After the mixture had cooled to room temperature, the absorbance of each solution was measured at 695 nm against a blank. Total antioxidant capacity was expressed as ascorbic acid equivalent.

4.11.2. Hydroxyl Radical Scavenging Activity Assay

The scavenging activity of seaweed polysaccharides against the hydroxyl radical was investigated using Fenton's reaction ($Fe^{2+} + H_2O_2 \rightarrow Fe^{3+} + OH^- + OH$). These results were expressed as inhibition rate. Hydroxyl radicals were generated using 3 mL sodium phosphate buffer (150 mM, pH 7.4), which contained 10 mM $FeSO_4.7H_2O$, 10 mM EDTA, 2 mM sodium salicylate, 30% H_2O_2 (200 mL) and varying polysaccharide concentrations. In the control, sodium phosphate buffer replaced H_2O_2. The solutions were incubated at 37 °C for 1 h, and the presence of the hydroxyl radical was detected by monitoring absorbance at 510 nm. Gallic acid was used as positive control.

4.11.3. Superoxide Radical Scavenging Activity Assay

This assay was based on the capacity of sulfated polysaccharides to inhibit the photochemical reduction of NBT in the riboflavin–light–NBT system. Each 3 mL of reaction mixture contained 50 mM phosphate buffer (pH 7.8), 13 mM methionine, 2 mM riboflavin, 100 mM EDTA, NBT (75 mM) and 1 mL sample solution. After the production of blue formazan, the increase in absorbance at 560 nm after 10 min illumination from a fluorescent lamp was determined. The entire reaction assembly was enclosed in a box lined with aluminum foil. Identical tubes with the reaction mixture were kept in the dark and served as blanks. Gallic acid was used as positive control.

4.11.4. Ferric Chelating

The ferrous ion chelating ability of samples was investigated using the following methodology: sulfated polysaccharides at different concentrations were applied with the reaction mixture, which contained $FeCl_2$ (0.05 mL, 2 mM) and ferrozine (0.2 mL, 5 mM). The mixture was shaken and incubated for 10 min at room temperature and absorbance of the mixture was measured at 562 nm against a blank. EDTA was used as positive control.

4.11.5. Cupric Chelating

Pyrocatechol violet, the reagent used in this assay, has the ability to associate with certain cations such as aluminum, copper, bismuth, and thorium. In the presence of chelating agents this combination is not formed, resulting in decreased staining. This reduction thus allows the estimation of the chelating activity of the copper ion from the fraction from *U. flabellum*. The test is performed in 96-well microplates with a reaction mixture containing different concentrations of samples (0.1–20 mg/mL), pyrocatechol violet (4 mM), and copper II sulfate pentahydrate (50 mg/mL). All wells were homogenized with the aid of a micropipette and the solution absorbance was measured at 632 nm. The ability of the samples in chelating the copper ion was calculated using the following equation:

$$(\text{Absorbance of blank}) - (\text{Absorbance of the sample})/(\text{Absorbance of the blank}) \times 100$$

4.12. Electrophoresis in Agarose Gel

Agarose gel electrophoresis of the acidic polysaccharides was performed in 0.6% agarose gel (7.5 cm × 10 cm × 0.2 cm thick) prepared in 0.05 M 1.3-diaminopropane acetate buffer pH 9.0, as previously described [15]. Aliquots of the polysaccharides (about 50 µg) were applied to the gel and subjected to electrophoresis. The gel was fixed with 0.1% cetyltrimethylammonium bromide solution for 2 h, dried, and stained for 15 min with 0.1% toluidine blue in 1% acetic acid in 50% ethanol. The gel was then destained with the same solution without the dye.

4.13. Statistical Analysis

All data were expressed as mean ± standard deviation of three observation ($n = 3$). Statistical analysis was done by one-way analysis of variance (ANOVA) followed by the Turkey-Kramer test. All tests were conducted on the SigmaPlot® (Systat software, San Jose, CA, USA). In all cases, statistical significance was set at $p < 0.05$.

5. Conclusions

We obtained six antioxidant sulfated polysaccharide-rich fractions from the green alga *U. flabellum*. These fractions mainly comprised heterogalactans, and were designated UF-0.3, UF-0.5, UF-0.6, UF-0.7, UF-1.0, and UF-2.0. None of the fractions exhibited cytotoxicity or inhibited 3T3 fibroblast proliferation. The four fractions that were assessed protected the cells from oxidative damage. UF-2.0 was the most effective in reducing oxidative stress when the cells were exposed to $CuSO4$; this can be attributed to the copper chelating ability of the fraction. The most effective fraction in mitigating oxidative stress in the presence of $FeSO4$ was UF-0.7. However, this effectiveness cannot be attributed solely to the ability of the fractions to chelate iron.

Our aims for future studies include identification of other mechanisms involved in mitigation of oxidative stress caused by compounds of iron and the role of sulfated polysaccharides in such mitigation. In addition, as UF-0.7 showed notable protective activity both in the presence of copper and iron, we intend to assess its effect in vivo to identify its role as a putative drug to be used for the treatment of diseases associated with elevated levels of copper and/or iron.

Acknowledgments: The authors wish to thank Conselho Nacional de Desenvolvimento Científico e Tecnológico-CNPq (National Council for Scientific and Technological Advancement, in loose translation), Coordenação de Aperfeiçoamento Pessoal de Nível Superior-CAPES (Higher Level Personal Development Coordination, in loose translation), Programa Nacional de Cooperação Acadêmica (PROCAD), Ciências do Mar/CAPES, and Ministério de Ciência, Tecnologia, Inovação e Comércio (MCTIC) (the Science and Technology Ministry in Brazil, in loose translation) for the financial support. Hugo Rocha is an honored researcher of the CNPq. The authors would like to thank the Department of Biochemistry at Universidade Federal do Rio Grande do Norte for letting us use the cell culture room. This research was presented at Programa de Pós-Graduação em Ciências da Saúde at Universidade Federal do Rio Grande do Norte, as part of the M.Sc. thesis of Fernando Presa.

Author Contributions: Fernando Bastos Presa prepared the samples. Fernando Bastos Presa and Maxsuell Lucas Mendes Marques performed the chemical analysis. Fernando Bastos Presa, Leonardo Thiago Duarte Barreto Nobre, Rony Lucas Silva Viana, Leandro Silva Costa and Maxsuell Lucas Mendes Marques performed tests with the 3T3-cells. Fernando Bastos Presa performed the antioxidant tests. Fernando Bastos Presa and Maxsuell Lucas Mendes Marques analyzed the data. Fernando Bastos Presa, Maxsuell Lucas Mendes Marques and Hugo Alexandre Oliveira Rocha wrote the paper. Leandro Silva Costa and Hugo Alexandre Oliveira Rocha funded and revised the paper.

Conflicts of Interest: The authors declare no conflict of interest.

References

1. Kremastinos, D.T.; Farmakis, D. Iron overload cardiomyopathy in clinical practice. *Contemp. Rev. Cardiovasc. Med.* **2011**, *124*, 2253–2263. [CrossRef]

2. Dong, Q.; Wu, Z. Advance in the pathogenesis and treatment of Wilson disease. *Transl. Neurodegener.* **2012**, *1*, 1–8. [CrossRef]

3. Dixon, S.J.; Stockwell, B.R. The role of iron and reactive oxygen species in cell death. *Nat. Chem. Biol.* **2014**, *10*, 9–17. [CrossRef]

4. Brewer, G.J. Novel therapeutic approaches to the treatment of Wilson's disease. *Expert Opin. Pharmacother.* **2006**, *7*, 317–324. [CrossRef]

5. Hansen, J.B.; Moen, I.W.; Mandrup-Poulsen, T. Iron: The hard player in diabetes pathophysiology. *Acta Physiol.* **2014**, *210*, 717–732. [CrossRef]

6. Campo, G.M.; D'Ascola, A.; Avenoso, A.; Campo, S.; Ferlazzo, A.M.; Micali, C.; Zanghí, L.; Calatroni, A. Glycosaminoglycans reduce oxidative damage induced by copper (Cu^{+2}), iron (Fe^{+2}) and hydrogen peroxide (H_2O_2) in human fibroblast cultures. *Glycoconj. J.* **2004**, *2*, 133–141. [CrossRef]

7. Negreiros, M.M.F.; Almeida-Lima, J.; Rocha, H.A.O. Sulfated Polysaccharides from Unusual Natural Sources. In *Sulfated Polysaccharides*, 1st ed.; Gama, M., Nader, H.B., Rocha, H.A.O., Eds.; Nova Science Publishers: New York, NY, USA, 2015; Volume 1, pp. 217–234, ISBN 978-1-63482-975-5.

8. Shao, P.; Chen, X.X.; Sun, P.L. In vitro antioxidant and antitumor activities of different sulfated polysaccharides isolated from three algae. *Int. J. Biol. Macromol.* **2013**, *62*, 155–161. [CrossRef]

9. Qi, H.; Zhang, Q.; Zhao, T.; Chen, R.; Zhang, H.; Niu, X.; LI, Z. Antioxidant activity of different sulfate content derivatives of polysaccharide extracted from *Ulva pertusa* (Chlorophyta) in vitro. *Int. J. Biol. Macromol.* **2005**, *4*, 15–37. [CrossRef]

10. Costa, M.S.S.P.; Costa, L.S.; Cordeiro, S.L.; Almeida-Lima, J.; Santos, N.D.; Magalhães, K.D.; Sabry, D.A.; Albuquerque, I.R.L.; Pereira, M.R.; Leite, E.L.; et al. Evalutaing the possible anticoagulant and antioxidant effects of sulfated polysaccharides from the tropical green alga *Caulerpa cupressoides* var. Flabellata. *J. Appl. Phycol.* **2012**, *24*, 1159–1167. [CrossRef]

11. Costa, L.S.; Fidelis, G.P.; Cordeiro, S.L.; Oliveira, R.M.; Sabry, D.A.; Câmara, R.B.; Nobre, L.T.; Costa, M.S.; Almeida-Lima, J.; Farias, E.H.; et al. Biological activities of sulfated polysaccharides from tropical seaweeds. *Biomed. Pharmacother.* **2010**, *64*, 21–28. [CrossRef]

12. Farias, E.H.; Pomin, V.H.; Valente, A.P.; Nader, H.B.; Rocha, H.A.; Mourão, P.A. A preponderantly 4-sulfated, 3-linked galactan from the green alga *Codium isthmocladum*. *Glycobiology* **2008**, *3*, 250–259. [CrossRef]

13. Arata, P.X.; Quintana, I.; Raffo, M.P.; Ciancia, M. Novel sulfated xylogalactoarabinans from green seaweed *Cladophora falklandica*: Chemical structure and action on the fibrin network. *Carbohydr. Polym.* **2016**, *154*, 139–150. [CrossRef]

14. Alves, A. Sulfated Polysaccharides from Green Seaweed. In *Sulfated Polysaccharides*, 1st ed.; Gama, M., Nader, H.B., Rocha, H.A.O., Eds.; Nova Science Publishers: New York, NY, USA, 2015; Volume 1, pp. 135–153, ISBN 978-1-63482-975-5.

15. Dietrich, C.P.; Dietrich, S.M. Electrophoretic behaviour of acidic mucopolysaccharides in diamine buffers. *Anal. Biochem.* **1976**, *70*, 645–647. [CrossRef]

16. Hayakawa, Y.; Hayashi, T.; Lee, J.; Srisomporn, P.; Maeda, M.; Ozawa, T.; Sakuragawa, N. Inhibition of thrombin by sulfated polysaccharides isolated from green algae. *Biochim. Biophys. Acta* **2000**, *1543*, 86–94. [CrossRef]

17. Wenjun Mao, W.; Zang, X.; Li, Y.; Zhang, H. Sulfated polysaccharides from marine green algae *Ulva conglobata* and their anticoagulant activity. *J. Appl.* **2006**, *18*, 9–14. [CrossRef]

18. Valko, M.; Leibfritz, D.; Moncol, J.; Cronin, M.T.; Mazur, M.; Telser, J. Free radicals and antioxidants in normal physiological functions and human disease. *Int. J. Biochem. Cell Biol.* **2007**, *39*, 44–84. [CrossRef]

19. Jomova, K.; Vondrakova, D.; Lawson, M.; Valko, M. Metals, oxidative stress and neurodegenerative disorders. *Mol. Cell. Biochem.* **2010**, *345*, 91–104. [CrossRef]

20. Nappi, A.J.; Vass, E. Comparative studies of enhanced iron-mediated production of hydroxyl radical by glutathione, cysteine, ascorbic acid, and selected catechols. *Biochim. Biophys. Acta* **1997**, *1336*, 295–301. [CrossRef]

21. Mak, W.; Hamid, N.; Liu, T.; Lu, J.; White, W.L. Fucoidan from New Zealand *Undaria pinnatifida*: Monthly variations and determination of antioxidant activities. *Carbohydr. Polym.* **2013**, *95*, 606–614. [CrossRef]

22. Melo, K.R.; Câmara, R.B.; Queiroz, M.F.; Vidal, A.A.; Lima, C.R.; Melo-Silveira, R.F.; Almeida-Lima, J.; Rocha, H.A. Evaluation of sulfated polysaccharides from the brown seaweed *Dictyopteris justii* as antioxidant agents and as inhibitors of the formation of calcium oxalate crystals. *Molecules* **2013**, *25*, 14543–14563. [CrossRef]

23. Galinari, E.; Almeida-Lima, J.; Macedo, G.R.; Mantovani, H.C.; Rocha, H.A. Antioxidant, antiproliferative, and immunostimulatory effects of cellwall-d-mannan fractions from *Kluyveromyces marxianu*. *Int. J. Biol. Macromol.* **2018**, *109*, 837–846. [CrossRef]

24. Oral, B.; Guney, M.; Demirin, H.; Ozguner, M.; Giray, S.G.; Take, G.; Mungan, T.; Altuntas, I. Endometrial damage and apoptosis in rats induced by dichlorvos and ameliorating effect of antioxidant vitamins E and C. *Reprod. Toxicol.* **2006**, *22*, 783–790. [CrossRef]

25. Knigth, J.A. Review: Free radicals, antioxidants, and the immune System. *Ann. Clin. Lab. Sci.* **2000**, *30*, 145–158.

26. Campo, G.M.; Avenoso, A.; Campo, S.; D'Ascola, A.; Traina, P.; Samà, D.; Calatroni, A. NF-kB and caspases are involved in the hyaluronan and chondroitin-4-sulphate-exerted antioxidant effect in fibroblast cultures exposed to oxidative stress. *J. Appl. Toxicol.* **2008**, *28*, 509–517. [CrossRef]

27. Dodgson, K.S.; Price, R.G. A note on the determination of the ester sulphate content of sulphated polysaccharides. *Biochem. J.* **1962**, *84*, 106–110.

28. Spector, J. Refinement of the coomassie blue method of protein quantification. A simple and linear spectrophotometric assay of 0.5 to 50 μg of protein. *Anal. Biochem.* **1978**, *86*, 142–143. [CrossRef]

29. Somogyi, M. Notes on sugar determination. *J. Biol. Chem.* **1952**, *195*, 19–23.

30. Rocha-Amorim, M.O.; Gomes, D.L.; Dantas, L.A.; Viana, R.L.S.; Chiquetti, S.C.; Almeida-Lima, J.; Silva Costa, L.; Rocha, H.A.O. Fucan-coated silver nanoparticles synthesized by a green method induce human renal adenocarcinoma cell death. *Int. J. Biol. Macromol.* **2016**, *93*, 57–65. [CrossRef]

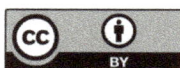

marine drugs

MDPI

Article

Fucoidan Inhibits Radiation-Induced Pneumonitis and Lung Fibrosis by Reducing Inflammatory Cytokine Expression in Lung Tissues

Hsin-Hsien Yu [1,2,†], Edward Chengchuan KO [3,4,5,†], Chia-Lun Chang [6,7], Kevin Sheng-Po Yuan [8], Alexander T. H. Wu [9], Yan-Shen Shan [1,10,*] and Szu-Yuan Wu [7,11,*]

[1] Institute of Clinical Medicine, College of Medicine, National Cheng Kung University, Tainan 701, Taiwan; klaus610@gmail.com

[2] Division of General Surgery, Department of Surgery, Wan Fang Hospital, Taipei Medical University, Taipei 116, Taiwan

[3] School of Dentistry, College of Dental Medicine, Kaohsiung Medical University, Kaohsiung 807, Taiwan; ko.edward.kaseizen@gmail.com

[4] Division of Oral and Maxillofacial Surgery, Kaohsiung Medical University Hospital, Kaohsiung 807, Taiwan

[5] Department of FUJISOFT Cartilage and Bone Regeneration, Tissue Engineering, The University of Tokyo, Tokyo 113-0033, Japan

[6] Department of Hemato-Oncology, Wan Fang Hospital, Taipei Medical University, Taipei 116, Taiwan; richardch9@hotmail.com

[7] Department of Internal Medicine, School of Medicine, College of Medicine, Taipei Medical University, Taipei 11031, Taiwan

[8] Department of Otorhinolaryngology, Wan Fang Hospital, Taipei Medical University, Taipei 116, Taiwan; dryuank@gmail.com

[9] Ph.D. Program for Translational Medicine, Taipei Medical University, Taipei 11031, Taiwan; chaw1211@tmu.edu.tw

[10] Department of Surgery, National Cheng Kung University Hospital, College of Medicine, National Cheng Kung University, Tainan 701, Taiwan

[11] Department of Radiation Oncology, Wan Fang Hospital, Taipei Medical University, Taipei 116, Taiwan

*   Correspondence: ysshan@mail.ncku.edu.tw (Y.-S.S.); szuyuanwu5399@gmail.com (S.-Y.W.)

†   These authors have contributed equally to this study.

Received: 5 July 2018; Accepted: 15 October 2018; Published: 19 October 2018

Abstract: Purpose: Radiotherapy is a crucial treatment approach for many types of cancer. Radiation pneumonitis (RP) is one of the major complications in chest irradiation. Fucoidan is a sulfated polysaccharide found mainly in various species of brown seaweed. Recent studies have demonstrated the anti-inflammatory effects of fucoidan. However, no study has reported a well-established prophylactic agent for RP. Therefore, we investigated the effects of fucoidan on RP and radiotherapy (RT)-induced lung fibrosis. **Materials and Methods**: We compared RP and RT-induced fibrosis in lung tissue specimens obtained from irradiated (10 Gy/shot) C57BL/6 mice with or without fucoidan administration (200 mg/kg/day, oral gavage for 14 days). The expression patterns of cytokines in the pleural fluid were determined using a cytokine array and confirmed through enzyme immunoassays. **Results**: Fucoidan administration attenuated RP and RT-induced fibrosis in lung tissues. Decreased neutrophil and macrophage accumulation was observed in irradiated lung tissues, and radiation-induced lung fibrosis, as demonstrated by Masson trichrome staining, was attenuated. We investigated the expression patterns of inflammatory cytokines in the irradiated lung pleural fluid through the protein array; results revealed that fucoidan administration changed the expression patterns of inflammatory cytokines in irradiated lung tissues. Furthermore, the expression levels of TIMP-1, CXCL1, MCP-1, MIP-2, and interleukin-1Ra were substantially enhanced in the pleural fluid, but fucoidan administration significantly reduced their expression. **Conclusions**: Fucoidan changes the expression patterns of inflammatory cytokines, which may consequently attenuate RP and RT-induced lung fibrosis.

Keywords: radiation pneumonitis; lung fibrosis; fucoidan; cytokine; macrophage; neutrophil

---

1. Introduction

Currently, radiotherapy (RT) is an important approach for treating tumors [1]. The treatment protocol can include curative, adjuvant, neoadjuvant, therapeutic, or palliative therapy, depending on the tumor type, location, and stage as well as the health status of patients [2,3]. Radiation pneumonitis (RP) is the acute manifestation of radiation-induced lung disease and is relatively common following RT for chest wall or intrathoracic malignancies [4]. The acute phase typically occurs between 4 and 12 weeks following the completion of the RT course; however, it may occur as early as 1 week after RT, particularly in patients receiving a high total dose or concurrent chemotherapy [5]. The late phase is characterized by lung fibrosis that occurs as early as 6 months following RT and can progressively continue for several years [6]. Typical symptoms include cough, dyspnea, low-grade fever, chest discomfort, and pleuritic pain. Moreover, the pathology of RP reflects an acute response of the lung to radiation and includes loss of type I pneumocytes and increased capillary permeability that result in interstitial and alveolar edema and the ingress of inflammatory cells into alveolar spaces. Immune-mediated lymphocytic alveolitis has been postulated as the underlying cause of changes in nonirradiated lung tissues [7,8]. Cytokines have been found to play crucial roles in RP and late RT-induced lung fibrosis [9–11].

Studies have indicated that preventing or treating RT-induced lung injury is difficult. Until now, no study has reported well-established prophylactic agents for RT-induced lung injury prevention or treatment. Patients who require chest RT have a risk of RP or lung fibrosis, which exerts acute or long-term effects. Therefore, it is necessary to identify an effective prophylactic agent that not only prevents RT-induced lung injury, but also guides the dose escalation of RT to achieve improved local control and overall survival.

A heparin-like molecule, referred to as fucoidan, containing high percentages of L-fucose and sulfated ester groups and small proportions of D-xylose, D-galactose, D-mannose, and glucuronic acid was found in the cell wall matrix of brown seaweed [12]. Various biological activities, such as antioxidant, anti-inflammatory, antiproliferative, anticancer, and proapoptotic activities, have been observed in brown seaweed [13–15]. Furthermore, radioprotective effects of fucoidan were observed in mice treated with total body irradiation [16]. The present study investigated the effects of fucoidan on RP and RT-induced lung fibrosis.

2. Material and Methods

2.1. Fucoidan Reagent

Fucoidan powder extracted from Sargassum hemiphyllum was obtained from Hi-Q Oligo-fucoidan, a commercial product provided by Hi-Q Marine Biotech International Ltd. (New Taipei City, Taiwan). Fucoidan powder or dextran powder (D9260; Sigma-Aldrich, St. Louis, MO, USA) was dissolved in double-distilled H2O and stirred at 25 °C for 30 min. The dissolved solution was filtered using 0.22-μm sterile filters (Millipore, Billerica, MA, USA). Fucoidan used in this study was obtained through the enzyme hydrolysis of original fucoidan. The average molecular weight, fucose content, and sulfate content of fucoidan used in this study were 0.8 KDa (92.1%), 210.9 ± 3.3 mmol/g, and $38.9\% \pm 0.4\%$ (w/w), respectively [17].

2.2. Animals and Grouping

Eight-week-old male C57BL/6 mice, weighing approximately 25 g, were used as experimental subjects. These mice were divided into four study groups: sham (mice not treated with lung irradiation but were immobilized), RT (mice treated with lung irradiation and administered double-distilled

H$_2$O; 200 µL/day, oral gavage for 14 days), RT + fucoidan (mice treated with lung irradiation and administered fucoidan; 200 mg/kg/day in 200 µL, oral gavage for 14 days), and fucoidan (mice administered fucoidan; 200 mg/kg/day in 200 µL, oral gavage for 14 days). RT + dextran (mice treated with lung irradiation and administered dextran; 200 mg/kg/day in 200 µL, oral gavage for 14 days), and fucoidan (mice administered fucoidan; 200 mg/kg/day in 200 µL, oral gavage for 14 days). In the fucoidan or dextran-receiving groups, fucoidan or dextran was administered through oral gavage for 3 days before RT; we defined the first day of fucoidan or dextran administration as day 1. RT was administered on day 3, and fucoidan or dextran was administered for 14 days. To obtain the lung tissue for neutrophil and macrophage identification and the pleural fluid, some mice were sacrificed on day 15. To obtain the lung tissue for fibrosis determination, some mice were sacrificed on day 31. Mice were inhalationally anesthetized with 5% isoflurane (2-chloro-2-(difluoromethoxy)-1,1,1-trifluoro-ethane) for 5 min and then placed in a CO$_2$ chamber. A fill rate of approximately 10% to 30% of the chamber volume per minute with 100% CO$_2$ was used, and mice were unconscious within 2–3 min. We maintained CO$_2$ flow for a minimum of 1 min after their respiration ceased. This study protocol was approved by the Institutional Animal Care and Use Committee at Wan Fang Hospital, Taipei Medical University (No. LAC-2015-0167). All animal experiments were performed in accord with relevant guidelines and regulations.

2.3. Mouse Lung Irradiation

C57BL/6 mice were immobilized using a customized harness that allowed for the exposure of the trunk along with the whole lung. Fluoroscopy and computed tomography were conducted to determine the position of the lung, design the radiation field, and calculate the dose distribution. The whole lung was irradiated with a rectangular field. The remainder of the body was shielded 5 half-value layers of lead. A linear accelerator (Elekta, 6-MV photon beam, Crawley, UK) was used to perform whole lung irradiation at 10 Gy.

2.4. Lung Tissue Dissection

Irradiated or sham C57/B6 mice were sacrificed at the aforementioned time points. Mice were anesthetized with 5% isoflurane, and their pleural fluid was withdrawn 30 s after administering 0.5 mL of normal saline intrapleurally by using a 23-gauge needle. The pleural fluid was then centrifuged at 3000 rpm for 10 min, and the supernatant was collected to perform cytokine analysis, ELISA, or functional assays. To avoid the damage caused by intrapleural injection, lung tissue samples were collected from another group of mice and subsequently embedded in paraffin for sectioning. To determine the expression of collagen I in the lung tissue, the freshly excised whole left lung lobe tissue was homogenized in liquid nitrogen. The total protein content of this tissue was extracted using a cell lysis buffer (Thermo Fisher Scientific, Waltham, MA, USA) and quantified using the Bio-Rad protein assay (Hercules, CA, USA).

2.5. Immunohistochemistry

The paraffin-embedded tissue slides were rehydrated in PBS for 15 min, and endogenous peroxidase activity was inhibited by 3% H$_2$O$_2$ or methanol for 10 min at room temperature. For blocking, 5% nonfat milk or PBS was added for 30 min at room temperature. The slides were incubated with an anti-F4/80 antibody or anti-Ly6G antibody or control IgG at 1:100 dilution for 16 h at 4 °C (F4/80 [C-7] is a mouse monoclonal antibody raised against amino acids 335–634 mapped within an extracellular domain of F4/80 of mouse origin; sc-377009; Santa Cruz Biotechnology; anti-Ly6G antibody is a monoclonal antibody NIMP-R14 is highly specific for murine Ly-6G [NIMP-R14]; (ab2557); Abcam). A peroxidase-conjugated secondary antibody was incubated for 1 h at room temperature and detected by immersing the slides in 0.06% 3,3′-diaminobenzidine tetrahydrochloride, followed by counterstaining with Gill Hematoxylin V.

2.6. Masson Trichrome Staining

Masson trichrome staining is widely used to study muscular pathologies, including tissue fibrosis and myofibroblasts, and also to detect and analyze myofibroblasts in lung biopsies [18,19]. Lung sections were stained with Masson Trichrome (Sigma-Aldrich, Saint Louis, MO, USA).

2.7. Real-Time Quantitative Reverse Transcription–Polymerase Chain Reaction

The mRNA expressions of Ly6G and F4/80 in the lung tissue were measured using a fluorescein real-time quantitative reverse transcription–polymerase chain reaction (qRT-PCR) detection system (Light Cycler DNA Master SYBR Green I; Roche Molecular Biochemicals, Indianapolis, IN, USA). Primer pairs used were as follows: GAPDH: 5'-GGGAAGGTGAAGGTCGG-3' and 5'-TGGACTCCACGACGTACTCAG-3'; Ly6G: 5'-TGGACTCTCACAGAAGCAAAG-3' and 5'-GCAGAGGTCTTCCTTCCAACA-3'; and F4/80: 5'-CTCTGTGGTCCCACCTTCAT-3' and 5'-GATGGCCAAGGATCTGAA AA-3'. The amplification program consisted of one cycle of initial incubation at 60 °C for 20 min, followed by 40 cycles of denaturation at 95 °C for 10 s, annealing at 55 °C for 10 s, and extension at 72 °C for 10 s. The relative mRNA level was calculated using the $2^{-\Delta\Delta Ct}$ method. The amount of indicated mRNA was normalized to that of GAPDH mRNA and presented in arbitrary units, with 1 U corresponding to the value of the sham group.

2.8. Cytokine Array

A mouse cytokine array (Ary006; Proteome Profiler, R&D Systems, Minneapolis, MN, USA) was used to analyze cytokine expression patterns in the pleural fluid. The pleural fluid was first mixed with a biotinylated detection antibody cocktail at room temperature for 1 h, and the array membrane was blocked with the blocking solution provided by the manufacturer. The membrane was then incubated with the samples overnight at 4 °C on a shaker. After washing, horseradish peroxidase-conjugated streptavidin was added to the membrane for 30 min at room temperature, and signal development was achieved by the addition of commercial chemiluminescence detection reagents. A digital imaging system (Bio Pioneer Tech Co., New Taipei City, Taiwan) was used to detect signals, which were further analyzed using the ImageJ program. The number of specimens, N, was 3 per experimental group, and a mean value was calculated.

2.9. Determination of TIMP-1, CXCL1, MCP-1, MIP-2, and Interleukin-1Ra

The protein lysate or serum levels of TIMP-1, CXCL1, MCP-1, MIP-2, and interleukin (IL)-1Ra were determined using enzyme immunoassay (EIA) kits (R&D Systems, Minneapolis, MN, USA). The protein levels of pro-collagen I alpha in the lung tissue lysate were determined using a mouse pro-collagen I alpha 1 ELISA kit (ab210579).

2.10. Functional Test of the Pleural Fluid for Type I Collagen Expression in Fibroblasts

NIH-3T3 cells were purchased from the American Type Culture Collection (Rockville, MD, USA). Cells are maintained in DMEM (Life Technologies, New York, NY, USA) supplemented with 10% (*vol/vol*) fetal bovine serum plus penicillin–streptomycin under sterile tissue culture conditions and cultured in a humidified atmosphere of 5% CO_2 and 95% air at 37 °C. NIH3T3 cells were cultured in 24-well plates until they reached a density of 1×10^5 cells/well. To prevent contamination of collagen in the pleural fluid, cells were treated with 100 μL of the pleural fluid obtained from different groups for 1 h. Subsequently, cells were washed, fresh medium was added, and the cell culture supernatant was collected after 24 h. The protein levels of type I collagen secreted into the cell culture supernatant were determined through ELISA.

2.11. Statistical Analysis

One-way ANOVA with Tukey's post hoc test was used to compare data among the groups. All statistical analyses were performed using SPSS for Windows, version 18.0 (SPSS Inc., Chicago, IL, USA). A *p* value of <0.05 was considered statistically significant.

3. Results

3.1. Fucoidan Attenuated RT-Induced Lung Fibrosis in Irradiated Mouse Lung Tissues

On the basis of the anti-inflammatory effect of fucoidan, we investigated its role in RT-induced lung fibrosis in a mouse model. Mice were divided into four groups, namely sham, RT, RT + fucoidan, and fucoidan, and sacrificed on day 31. We first determined pulmonary fibrosis in each group through Masson trichrome staining (Figure 1, left panel). Type I collagen, which is the major component of pulmonary fibrosis, is encoded by the COL1A1 gene. The COL1A1 gene produces a component of type I collagen, named pro-collagen 1 alpha. Thus, the whole left lobe of the lung was homogenized to determine the pro-collagen 1 alpha level through ELISA (Figure 1, right panel). The results of ELISA revealed increased collagen deposition in the RT group and attenuated collagen deposition in the RT + fucoidan group. The quantitative results of pro-collagen 1 alpha demonstrated that RT significantly enhanced collagen formation in the lung tissue (0.92 ± 0.05 mg/g in the sham group vs. 3.22 ± 0.39 mg/g in the RT group) and fucoidan administration significantly reduced the collagen level in the RT + fucoidan group (1.83 ± 0.23 mg/g). These results indicated that fucoidan attenuated RT-induced lung fibrosis in irradiated mouse lung tissues.

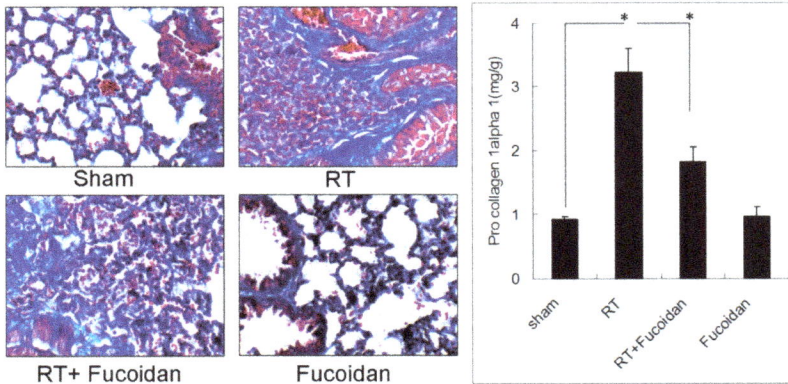

Figure 1. Effects of fucoidan on lung fibrosis in irradiated mouse lung tissues. (**Left** panel): mice from indicated groups were sacrificed on day 31. Representative images of Masson trichrome staining of mouse lung tissues (400×). (**Right** panel): the whole left lobe of the lung of each mouse in each group was homogenized to determine the pro-collagen 1 alpha level through ELISA. N = 5/group. * *p* < 0.05 by one-way ANOVA with Tukey's post hoc test.

3.2. Fucoidan Reduced Neutrophil and Macrophage Infiltration in Irradiated Lung Tissues

Lung fibrosis is a sequential effect of inflammation. To address the specific effect of Fucoidan, dextran, which is a complex branched glucan is used as polysaccharide control. To observe the phenomenon of neutrophil and macrophage infiltration in lung tissue specimens, mice were divided into four study groups, namely sham, RT, RT + fucoidan, and RT + dextran, and sacrificed on day 15. A part of the lung tissue of each mouse was dissected to prepare paraffin-embedded sections. Neutrophil infiltration was determined through Ly6G antibody staining, which is a specific marker for mouse neutrophils are shown in Figure 2 (left panels). Macrophage infiltration in paraffin-embedded lung tissues was identified through F4/80 antibody staining, which is a specific marker for mouse macrophages (Figure 3, left panels). The whole left lobe of the lung of each mouse in each group was homogenized for use in qRT-PCR performed to determine the expression levels of Ly6G and F4/80, which are specific markers for neutrophils (Figure 2, right panel) and macrophages (Figure 3, right panel), respectively. The quantitative results of Ly6G and F4/80 mRNA demonstrated increased neutrophil (1-fold in the sham group vs. 16.8 ± 4.8-fold in the RT group) and macrophage (1-fold in the sham group vs. 4.8 ± 1.6-fold in the RT group) infiltration in the lung tissues of the RT group. However, the infiltration of neutrophils (7.74 ± 4.01-fold) and macrophages (1.94 ± 0.54-fold) significantly decreased in the RT + fucoidan group but not in RT + dextran group. Meanwhile, Fucoidan administration alone did not change the levels of neutrophil and macrophage infiltration in lung tissues (data not show).

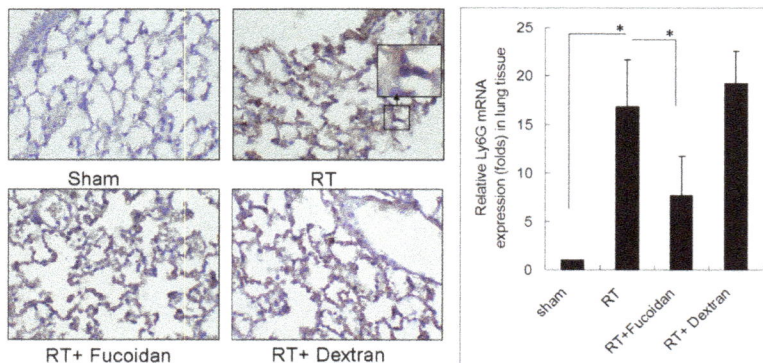

Figure 2. Effects of fucoidan on neutrophil infiltration in irradiated mouse lung tissues. (**Left** panel): mice from indicated groups were sacrificed on day 15. A representative image of neutrophil infiltration in lung tissues ($400\times$). (**Right** panel): the whole left lobe of the lung of each mouse in each group was homogenized for use in qRT-PCR performed for determining the expression level of Ly6G. N = 5/group. * $p < 0.05$ by one-way ANOVA with Tukey's post hoc test.

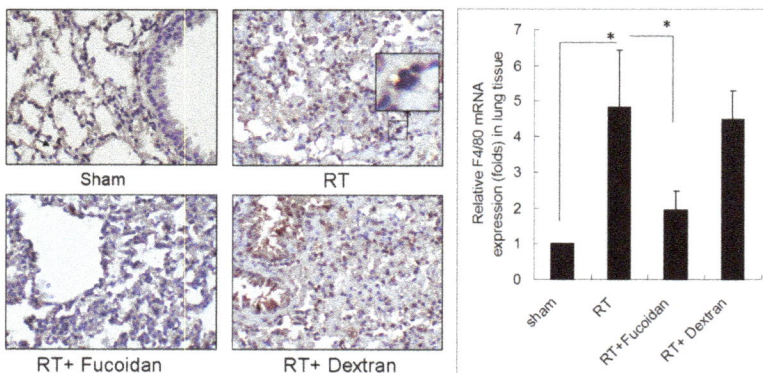

Figure 3. Effects of fucoidan on F4/80 macrophage infiltration in irradiated mouse lung tissues. (**Left** panel): mice from indicated groups were sacrificed on day 15. A representative image of F4/80 macrophage infiltration in lung tissues ($400\times$). (**Right** panel): the whole left lobe of the lung of each mouse in each group was homogenized for use in qRT-PCR performed for determining the expression level of F4/80. N = 5/group. * $p < 0.05$ by one-way ANOVA with Tukey's post hoc test.

3.3. Fucoidan Reduced Cytokine Expression in the Pleural Fluid Obtained from Irradiated Mice

Cytokine expression may reflect the status of inflammation. To examine the expression of cytokines in the lung tissue, mice were divided into four study groups, namely sham, RT, RT + fucoidan, and fucoidan, and sacrificed on day 15. The pleural fluid was collected to analyze the expression patterns of inflammatory cytokines by using a cytokine array. The images of the cytokine array (Figure 4, upper panel) and their corresponding quantitative results demonstrated that fucoidan administration changed the expression patterns of inflammatory cytokines in the pleural fluid obtained from irradiated mice (Figure 4, lower panel). The top five cytokines that were significantly induced in the pleural fluid of the irradiated group than in that of the sham group are as follows: TIMP-1 (3.71 ± 0.11-fold), CXCL1 (4.32 ± 0.12-fold), MCP-1 (4.27 ± 0.13-fold), MIP-2 (13.71 ± 0.14-fold), and IL-1Ra (3.37 ± 0.1-fold). Furthermore, they were significantly reduced in RT + fucoidan group. Additionally, TREM-1 was also induced in the pleural fluid of the irradiated group than in that of the sham group (2.27 ± 0.11-fold) and it was reduced in RT + fucoidan group. On the other hand, by comparing with sham group, the quantitative result revealed that SDF-1/CXCL12 (2.57 ± 0.13-fold) and IL-16 (1.93 ± 0.1-fold) were induced in the pleural fluid of the fucoidan administration only group. However, the expression of SDF-1/CXCL12 (0.37 ± 0.12-fold) and IL-16 (0.68 ± 0.08-fold) in RT + fucoidan group were low.

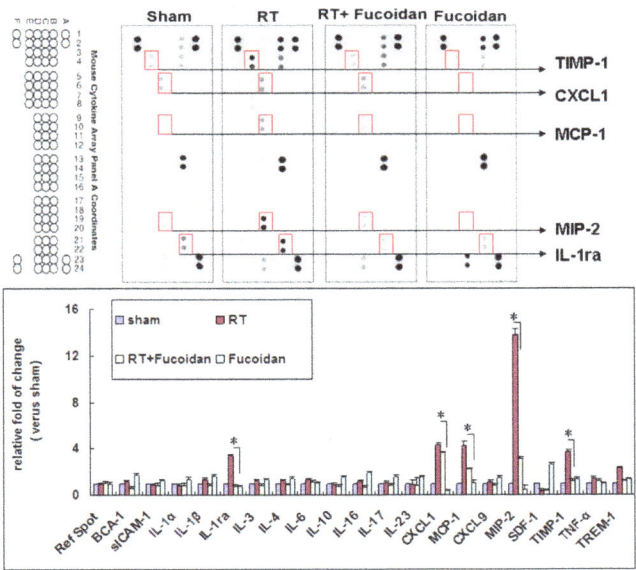

Figure 4. Effects of fucoidan on cytokine expression in the pleural fluid obtained from irradiated mice. (**Upper** panel): pleural fluid was collected from the mice of indicated groups on day 15. Representative image of the cytokine array of pleural fluids. Five spots with obvious changes are indicated. (**Lower** panel): quantitative results of cytokine spots. N = 3/group.

3.4. Fucoidan Reduced TIMP-1, CXCL1, MCP-1, MIP-2, and IL-1Ra Expression in the Pleural Fluid Obtained from Irradiated Mice

On the basis of the findings of the cytokine array described in Figure 4, we chose the following top five cytokines that were significantly induced in the sham group than in the RT groups: TIMP-1, CXCL1, MCP-1, MIP-2, and IL-1Ra. We determined the concentrations of these cytokines in the pleural fluid of mice in each group through EIA. The results revealed that the expression levels of TIMP-1 (203.1 ± 84.8 ng/mL in the sham group vs. 509.7 ± 151.1 ng/mL in the RT group; Figure 5A), CXCL1 (42.5 ± 17.9

pg/mL in the sham group vs. 145.8 ± 45 pg/mL in the RT group; Figure 5B), MCP-1 (28.6 ± 6.4 pg/mL in the sham group vs. 246.5 ± 80.4 pg/mL in the RT group; Figure 5C), MIP-2 (31.6 ± 16.8 pg/mL in the sham group vs. 143.2 ± 42.6 pg/mL in the RT group; Figure 5D), and IL-1Ra (98.4 ± 45.3 in the sham group vs. 1319.4 ± 203.4 μg/mL in the RT group; Figure 5E) were significantly enhanced in the collected pleural fluid. However, in the RT + fucoidan group, the levels of TIMP-1 (223.1 ± 30.7 ng/mL), CXCL1 (73.3 ± 26.4 pg/mL), MCP-1 (146.4 ± 30.8 pg/mL), MIP-2 (55 ± 27.3 pg/mL), and IL-1Ra (474.4 ± 146.7 μg/mL) were significantly decreased. In order to examine the effect of the cytokines induced by RT in the pleural fluid on fibroblasts and to assess fibrosis induction capability, NIH-3T3 cells, which is a well-known mouse fibroblast cell line, were treated with the pleural fluid obtained from mice in the sham, RT, RT + fucoidan, and fucoidan groups. The pro-collagen 1 alpha level in the cell culture supernatant was determined through ELISA (Figure 5F). The results revealed that, compared with the sham group, the pleural fluid obtained from mice in the RT group significantly increased the type I collagen level in the culture supernatant of NIH-3T3 cells (29.9 ± 6.9 ng/mL in the sham group vs. 70.6 ± 18.4 ng/mL in the RT group). However, compared with the RT group, the type I collagen level was decreased in the cell culture supernatant of NIH-3T3 cells treated with the pleural fluid obtained from mice in the RT + fucoidan group (42.8 ± 9.3 ng/mL).

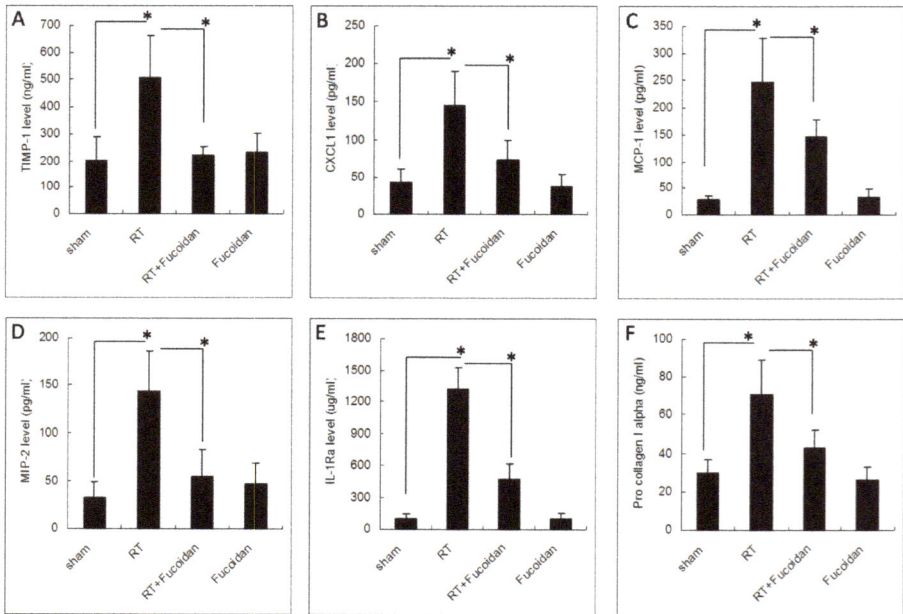

Figure 5. Effects of fucoidan on cytokine levels in the pleural fluid obtained from irradiated mice. The pleural fluid was collected from the mice of indicated groups on day 15. The expression levels of (**A**) TIMP-1, (**B**) CXCL1, (**C**) MCP-1, (**D**) MIP-2, and (**E**) IL-1ra were determined through enzyme immunoassays. Data are compared between indicated groups. * $p < 0.05$. N = 10/group. (**F**) NIH-3T3 cells were treated with the pleural fluid obtained from mice in the sham, RT, RT + fucoidan, and fucoidan groups for 1 h prior to the addition of fresh culture medium and then incubated for another 24 h. The cell culture supernatant was collected for determining the type I collagen level through ELISA. * $p < 0.05$. N = 6/group by one-way ANOVA with Tukey's post hoc test.

This study demonstrated that fucoidan administration in irradiated mice attenuated cytokine (TIMP-1, CXCL1, MCP-1, MIP-2, and IL-1Ra) expression in the collected pleural fluid and reduced pleural fluid-induced collagen expression in fibroblasts, which were correlated with the reduction of neutrophil and macrophage infiltration in lung tissues; macrophage and neutrophil infiltration may lead to RP and RT-induced lung fibrosis (Figure 6). This result may facilitate the design of fucoidan-based therapeutic approaches for preventing RP in clinical practice.

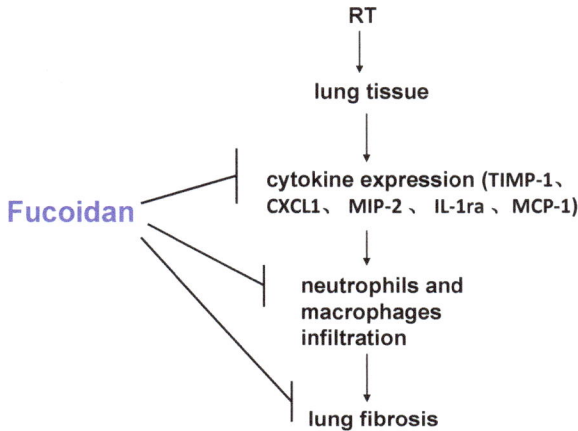

RT

↓

lung tissue

↓

Fucoidan

cytokine expression (TIMP-1、CXCL1、 MIP-2 、 IL-1ra 、 MCP-1)

↓

neutrophils and macrophages infiltration

↓

lung fibrosis

Figure 6. Schematic of possible molecular mechanisms underlying the preventive effects of fucoidan on radiotherapy (RT)-induced lung fibrosis mediated through the reduction of neutrophil and macrophage infiltration and alteration in cytokine expression patterns in lung tissues.

4. Discussion

According to a clinical description, RP occurs in the latent period. However, a molecular biology study revealed a cascade of events occurring immediately after injury and continuing up to the overall occurrence of clinical symptoms such as cough, dyspnea, low-grade fever, chest discomfort, and pleuritic pain [11]. Oxidative stress may cause DNA-damaging injuries; under such conditions, the immediate pulmonary response to radiation-induced injury is similar to many conventional wound healing responses. However, it remains unclear why radiation-induced lung injury is not completely repaired and resolved, with lung tissues consequently entering a progressive and dysregulated process that concludes in the late stage of RP and lung fibrosis. These injuries are now considered to be the result of a complex, structural interaction between multiple cell types, which is initiated and perpetuated through intercell and intracell signaling transduction pathways [20].

A previous study [21] investigated the tissue distribution of 100–200 mg/kg/day of fucoidan after intragastric administration in rats and reported considerable heterogeneity. Fucoidan preferentially accumulated in the kidneys (AUC0-t = 10.74 µg·h/g and Cmax = 1.23 µg/g after 5 h), spleen (AUC0-t = 6.89 µg·h/g and Cmax = 0.78 µg/g after 3 h), and liver (AUC0-t = 3.26 µg·h/g and Cmax = 0.53 µg/g after 2 h) and showed relatively long absorption time and extended circulation in the blood, with a mean residence time of 6.79 h. Although data regarding the fucoidan concentration in the lungs are not available, a study showed the anticancer effect of fucoidan on the lung tissue in vivo [22]. We did not perform a dose-dependent study before. The oral gavage dose administered in the current study was based on the dose suggested in previous studies (200 mg/kg) [23–25]. In addition, lung fibrosis is a sequential effect of inflammation. Because fucoidan may attenuate RT-induced inflammation and then reduce lung fibrosis, we examined the effects of fucoidan treatment only for 2 weeks, rather than for 3–4 weeks. We evaluated the phenomena of neutrophil and macrophage infiltration in lung tissue specimens.

RT techniques applied to patients with thorax-related malignancies have resulted in increased lung morbidity and mortality [26–30]. Such therapies involved the exposure of large areas of the heart or lungs to high radiation doses [2–4,29]. Although new treatment techniques have reduced both the dose of RT and the area of the heart or lungs exposed to the RT field, it is not clear whether the risk of late complications has been reduced in magnitude or has been merely delayed with regard to the onset time [27–30]. RT doses to the chest field, such as in breast, esophageal, or lung cancer, might be usually limited by lung or heart tolerance [26–29]. Furthermore, improved local control or overall survival through RT dose escalation is difficult because of the intolerance of normal tissues [26–29]. After a long-term follow-up, the grade of acute radiation-induced injury can often escalate to late radiation-induced injury, resulting in long-term RT-related complications [31]. In addition, similar to other organs, recovery from the acute effects of RT in the lungs does not always correlate with the prevention of late critical effects, including fibrosis, which contribute to organ failure [31]. An interventional agent, such as fucoidan, that can protect normal organ tissues from the acute and late effects of RT is crucial. The possibility of dose escalation for improved local control is important [32]. However, RT-induced toxicity in organs, such as the lungs, heart, or gastrointestinal tract, would be problematic in dose escalation because of the intolerance of normal tissues to RT [26–29]. Until now, no prospective controlled studies have evaluated the efficacy of any preventive drugs or therapies for RP in humans. This study is the first to evaluate the preventive effects of fucoidan on RP and RT-induced lung fibrosis.

In the present study, fucoidan attenuated RT-induced lung fibrosis in irradiated mouse lung tissues on day 31 (Figure 1). Radiation-induced lung injury results from the combination of direct cytotoxicity on normal lung tissues, and more importantly, from the development of fibrosis triggered by radiation-induced cellular signal transduction. The cytotoxic effects are mainly caused by DNA damage that leads to clonogenic death of normal lung epithelial cells, in addition to apoptotic pathways induced by radiation. Fucoidan significantly reduced neutrophil and macrophage infiltration in irradiated mouse lung tissues (Figures 2 and 3). A previous study reported that macrophages may also be present within the alveolar space; these macrophages are migratory cells from the bone marrow and act as a source of numerous cytokines, including IL-6 and TNF-α, to the lungs [33]. In our study, fucoidan attenuated RP and RT-induced lung fibrosis by reducing neutrophil and macrophage infiltration (Figure 6).

Several cytokines are upregulated following lung irradiation and together mediate the corresponding pathological changes. A previous clinical study demonstrated that RT induced the expression of transforming growth factor-beta 1 (TGF-β1), which induced fibroblast collagen deposition [34]. The plasma TGF-β1 level at the end of an RT course was observed to be a predictor of the risk of pneumonitis [34]. However, a subsequent clinical trial revealed no predictable pattern of TGF-β1 changes in individuals with and without radiation-induced lung injury [35]. The proinflammatory cytokines tumor necrosis factor-alpha (TNF-α) and IL-1α have been observed to be upregulated immediately following irradiation. The IL-6 concentration increases following RT, and an elevated pretreatment plasma IL-6 concentration has been shown to be correlated with an increased risk of radiation-induced lung injury [11,36]. However, in this study, we observed no significant differences in IL-1α, TNFα, or IL-6 levels between the sham and RT groups (Figure 4). The discrepancies in results might be due to different sites or the timing of sample collection in different studies. In our study, we collected the pleural fluid from mice of indicated groups on day 15, whereas in previous studies, samples were obtained from human plasma irradiated on day 1 [10,11,35,36]. In our study, the levels of TIMP-1, CXCL1, MCP-1, MIP-2, and IL-1ra were elevated in irradiated mice, which were reduced by fucoidan on day 15. The levels of TIMP-1, CXCL1, MCP-1, MIP-2, and IL-1ra were also determined through EIAs (Figure 5). Fucoidan reduced the expression of TIMP-1, CXCL1, MCP-1, MIP-2, and IL-1ra in the pleural fluid obtained from irradiated mice on day 15. The decreased expression of TIMP-1, CXCL1, MCP-1, MIP-2, and IL-1ra in the pleural fluid obtained from irradiated mice on day 15 was proportional to RT-induced lung fibrosis in mice from the indicated groups that were sacrificed on day 31 (Figure 1). In our study, the increased expression of TIMP-1, CXCL1, MCP-1, MIP-2, and IL-1ra was strongly associated with RT-induced lung fibrosis through the induction of alternatively activated macrophages and neutrophils [37–45]. In our current animal model, the pleural fluid was collected on day 15, and mice were sacrificed on day 31. These findings are consistent with late RT-induced lung injuries, such as lung fibrosis (Figure 1). The present results indicated that fucoidan might attenuate RT-induced lung fibrosis by reducing inflammatory cytokine expression and macrophage and neutrophil infiltration. In addition, the mechanism and role of fucoidan on the SDF-1/CXCL12 and IL-16 expression in normal lung tissue need to be further investigated.

Figure 6 presents a brief schematic of the possible molecular mechanism underlying the preventive effects of fucoidan on RT-induced lung fibrosis mediated through the reduction of inflammatory cytokine expression and neutrophil and macrophage infiltration in lung tissues. The strength of our study is that it is the first study to demonstrate the preventive effects of fucoidan on RP and RT-induced lung fibrosis. This finding can be considered in future clinical practice and randomized controlled studies. Therefore, to obtain crucial information on population specificity and disease occurrence, a large-scale randomized trial comparing the effects of fucoidan on carefully selected patients receiving chest irradiation is essential.

5. Conclusions

In our study, fucoidan changed the expression patterns of inflammatory cytokines, which may consequently attenuate RP and RT-induced lung fibrosis. Fucoidan can be a potential therapeutic agent for RP attenuation or prevention.

Author Contributions: Conception and design: S.-Y.W. Financial support: Taipei Medical University and Wan Fang Hospital (107-swf-08). Collection and assembly of data: E.C.K., C.-L.C., H.-H.Y., Y.-S.S., K.S.-P.Y., A.T.H.W. and S.-Y.W. Data analysis and interpretation: E.C.K., C.-L.C., H.-H.Y., Y.-S.S. and S.-Y.W. Administrative support: S.-Y.W. Manuscript writing: All authors. Final approval of manuscript: All authors.

Funding: Taipei Medical University and Wan Fang Hospital.

Acknowledgments: Taipei Medical University and Wan Fang Hospital (107-swf-08).

Conflicts of Interest: The authors have no potential conflicts of interest to declare. The datasets supporting the study conclusions are included within the manuscript.

Abbreviations

RT	Radiotherapy
RP	Radiation Pneumonitis
H&E	Hematoxylin and Eosin
EIAs	Enzyme Immunoassays
DAKO	Diaminobenzidine Tetrahydrochloride
ACEI	Angiotensin-Converting Enzyme Inhibitor
TGF-β1	Transforming Growth Factor-Beta 1
TNF-α	Tumor Necrosis Factor-Alpha
IL-1α	Interleukin 1-Alpha
IL-6	Interleukin 6

References

1. McDonald, S.; Rubin, P.; Phillips, T.L.; Marks, L.B. Injury to the lung from cancer therapy: Clinical syndromes, measurable endpoints, and potential scoring systems. *Int. J. Radiat. Oncol. Biol. Phys.* **1995**, *31*, 1187–1203. [CrossRef]
2. Morgan, G.W.; Breit, S.N. Radiation and the lung: A reevaluation of the mechanisms mediating pulmonary injury. *Int. J. Radiat. Oncol. Biol. Phys.* **1995**, *31*, 361–369. [CrossRef]
3. Marks, L.B.; Bentzen, S.M.; Deasy, J.O.; Kong, F.M.; Bradley, J.D.; Vogelius, I.S.; El Naqa, I.; Hubbs, J.L.; Lebesque, J.V.; Timmerman, R.D.; et al. Radiation dose-volume effects in the lung. *Int. J. Radiat. Oncol. Biol. Phys.* **2010**, *76*, S70–S76. [CrossRef] [PubMed]

4. Marks, L.B.; Yorke, E.D.; Jackson, A.; Ten Haken, R.K.; Constine, L.S.; Eisbruch, A.; Bentzen, S.M.; Nam, J.; Deasy, J.O. Use of normal tissue complication probability models in the clinic. *Int. J. Radiat. Oncol. Biol. Phys.* **2010**, *76*, S10–S19. [CrossRef] [PubMed]

5. Lingos, T.I.; Recht, A.; Vicini, F.; Abner, A.; Silver, B.; Harris, J.R. Radiation pneumonitis in breast cancer patients treated with conservative surgery and radiation therapy. *Int. J. Radiat. Oncol. Biol. Phys.* **1991**, *21*, 355–360. [CrossRef]

6. Rubin, P.; Casseratt, G.W.; Saunders, W. Respiratory system. In *Clinical Radiation Pathology*, 3rd ed.; W.B. Saunders: Philadelphia, PA, USA, 1968; pp. 423–470.

7. Kwa, S.L.; Lebesque, J.V.; Theuws, J.C.; Marks, L.B.; Munley, M.T.; Bentel, G.; Oetzel, D.; Spahn, U.; Graham, M.V.; Drzymala, R.E.; et al. Radiation pneumonitis as a function of mean lung dose: An analysis of pooled data of 540 patients. *Int. J. Radiat. Oncol. Biol. Phys.* **1998**, *42*, 1–9. [CrossRef]

8. Graham, M.V.; Purdy, J.A.; Emami, B.; Harms, W.; Bosch, W.; Lockett, M.A.; Perez, C.A. Clinical dose-volume histogram analysis for pneumonitis after 3D treatment for non-small cell lung cancer (NSCLC). *Int. J. Radiat. Oncol. Biol. Phys.* **1999**, *45*, 323–329. [CrossRef]

9. Rubin, P.; Johnston, C.J.; Williams, J.P.; McDonald, S.; Finkelstein, J.N. A perpetual cascade of cytokines postirradiation leads to pulmonary fibrosis. *Int. J. Radiat. Oncol. Biol. Phys.* **1995**, *33*, 99–109. [CrossRef]

10. Anscher, M.S.; Kong, F.M.; Marks, L.B.; Bentel, G.C.; Jirtle, R.L. Changes in plasma transforming growth factor beta during radiotherapy and the risk of symptomatic radiation-induced pneumonitis. *Int. J. Radiat. Oncol. Biol. Phys.* **1997**, *37*, 253–258. [CrossRef]

11. Chen, Y.; Williams, J.; Ding, I.; Hernady, E.; Liu, W.; Smudzin, T.; Finkelstein, J.N.; Rubin, P.; Okunieff, P. Radiation pneumonitis and early circulatory cytokine markers. *Semin. Radiat. Oncol.* **2002**, *12*, 26–33. [CrossRef] [PubMed]

12. Senthilkumar, K.; Manivasagan, P.; Venkatesan, J.; Kim, S.K. Brown seaweed fucoidan: Biological activity and apoptosis, growth signaling mechanism in cancer. *Int. J. Biol. Macromol.* **2013**, *60*, 366–374. [CrossRef] [PubMed]

13. Atashrazm, F.; Lowenthal, R.M.; Woods, G.M.; Holloway, A.F.; Dickinson, J.L. Fucoidan and cancer: A multifunctional molecule with anti-tumor potential. *Mar. Drugs* **2015**, *13*, 2327–2346. [CrossRef] [PubMed]

14. Kwak, J.Y. Fucoidan as a marine anticancer agent in preclinical development. *Mar. Drugs* **2014**, *12*, 851–870. [CrossRef] [PubMed]

15. Wu, S.Y.; Wu, A.T.; Yuan, K.S.; Liu, S.H. Brown seaweed fucoidan inhibits cancer progression by dual regulation of mir-29c/ADAM12 and miR-17-5p/PTEN axes in human breast cancer cells. *J. Cancer* **2016**, *7*, 2408–2419. [CrossRef] [PubMed]

16. Lee, J.; Kim, J.; Moon, C.; Kim, S.H.; Hyun, J.W.; Park, J.W.; Shin, T. Radioprotective effects of fucoidan in mice treated with total body irradiation. *Phytother. Res.* **2008**, *22*, 1677–1681. [CrossRef] [PubMed]

17. Hwang, P.A.; Phan, N.N.; Lu, W.J.; Ngoc Hieu, B.T.; Lin, Y.C. Low-molecular-weight fucoidan and high-stability fucoxanthin from brown seaweed exert prebiotics and anti-inflammatory activities in Caco-2 cells. *Food Nutr. Res.* **2016**, *60*, 32033. [CrossRef] [PubMed]

18. Szapiel, S.V.; Elson, N.A.; Fulmer, J.D.; Hunninghake, G.W.; Crystal, R.G. Bleomycin-induced interstitial pulmonary disease in the nude, athymic mouse. *Am. Rev. Respir. Dis.* **1979**, *120*, 893–899. [PubMed]

19. Moore, B.B.; Hogaboam, C.M. Murine models of pulmonary fibrosis. *Am. J. Physiol. Lung Cell Mol. Physiol.* **2008**, *294*, L152–L160. [CrossRef] [PubMed]

20. Folkman, J.; Camphausen, K. Cancer. What does radiotherapy do to endothelial cells? *Science* **2001**, *293*, 227–228. [CrossRef] [PubMed]

21. Pozharitskaya, O.N.; Shikov, A.N.; Faustova, N.M.; Obluchinskaya, E.D.; Kosman, V.M.; Vuorela, H.; Makarov, V.G. Pharmacokinetic and tissue distribution of fucoidan from fucus vesiculosus after oral administration to rats. *Mar. Drugs* **2018**, *16*, 132. [CrossRef] [PubMed]

22. Hsu, H.Y.; Lin, T.Y.; Wu, Y.C.; Tsao, S.M.; Hwang, P.A.; Shih, Y.W.; Hsu, J. Fucoidan inhibition of lung cancer in vivo and in vitro: Role of the Smurf2-dependent ubiquitin proteasome pathway in TGFbeta receptor degradation. *Oncotarget* **2014**, *5*, 7870–7885. [CrossRef] [PubMed]

23. Chen, L.M.; Liu, P.Y.; Chen, Y.A.; Tseng, H.Y.; Shen, P.C.; Hwang, P.A.; Hsu, H.L. Oligo-fucoidan prevents IL-6 and CCL2 production and cooperates with p53 to suppress ATM signaling and tumor progression. *Sci. Rep.* **2017**, *7*, 11864. [CrossRef] [PubMed]

24. Chen, C.H.; Sue, Y.M.; Cheng, C.Y.; Chen, Y.C.; Liu, C.T.; Hsu, Y.H.; Hwang, P.A.; Huang, N.J.; Chen, T.H. Oligo-fucoidan prevents renal tubulointerstitial fibrosis by inhibiting the CD44 signal pathway. *Sci. Rep.* **2017**, *7*, 40183. [CrossRef] [PubMed]

25. Tsai, H.L.; Tai, C.J.; Huang, C.W.; Chang, F.R.; Wang, J.Y. Efficacy of low-molecular-weight fucoidan as a supplemental therapy in metastatic colorectal cancer patients: A double-blind randomized controlled trial. *Mar. Drugs* **2017**, *15*, 122. [CrossRef] [PubMed]

26. Bradley, J.D.; Paulus, R.; Komaki, R.; Masters, G.; Blumenschein, G.; Schild, S.; Bogart, J.; Hu, C.; Forster, K.; Magliocco, A.; et al. Standard-dose versus high-dose conformal radiotherapy with concurrent and consolidation carboplatin plus paclitaxel with or without cetuximab for patients with stage IIIA or IIIB non-small-cell lung cancer (RTOG 0617): A randomised, two-by-two factorial phase 3 study. *Lancet Oncol.* **2015**, *16*, 187–199. [PubMed]

27. Wang, K.; Eblan, M.J.; Deal, A.M.; Lipner, M.; Zagar, T.M.; Wang, Y.; Mavroidis, P.; Lee, C.B.; Jensen, B.C.; Rosenman, J.G.; et al. Cardiac toxicity after radiotherapy for stage III non-small-cell lung cancer: Pooled analysis of dose-escalation trials delivering 70 to 90 Gy. *J. Clin. Oncol.* **2017**, *35*, 1387–1394. [CrossRef] [PubMed]

28. Speirs, C.K.; DeWees, T.A.; Rehman, S.; Molotievschi, A.; Velez, M.A.; Mullen, D.; Fergus, S.; Trovo, M.; Bradley, J.D.; Robinson, C.G. Heart dose is an independent dosimetric predictor of overall survival in locally advanced non-small cell lung cancer. *J. Thorac. Oncol.* **2017**, *12*, 293–301. [CrossRef] [PubMed]

29. Dess, R.T.; Sun, Y.; Matuszak, M.M.; Sun, G.; Soni, P.D.; Bazzi, L.; Murthy, V.L.; Hearn, J.W.D.; Kong, F.M.; Kalemkerian, G.P.; et al. Cardiac events after radiation therapy: Combined analysis of prospective multicenter trials for locally advanced non-small-cell lung cancer. *J. Clin. Oncol.* **2017**, *35*, 1395–1402. [CrossRef] [PubMed]

30. Jones, J.M.; Ribeiro, G.G. Mortality patterns over 34 years of breast cancer patients in a clinical trial of post-operative radiotherapy. *Clin. Radiol.* **1989**, *40*, 204–208. [CrossRef]

31. Epperly, M.; Bray, J.; Kraeger, S.; Zwacka, R.; Engelhardt, J.; Travis, E.; Greenberger, J. Prevention of late effects of irradiation lung damage by manganese superoxide dismutase gene therapy. *Gene Ther.* **1998**, *5*, 196–208. [CrossRef] [PubMed]

32. Morganti, A. Higher-dose radiotherapy ups survival in pancreatic cancer. In Proceedings of the European Society for Radiotherapy & Oncology, Vienna, Austria, 15 May 2017.

33. Chen, G.; Lin, S.C.; Chen, J.; He, L.; Dong, F.; Xu, J.; Han, S.; Du, J.; Entman, M.L.; Wang, Y. CXCL16 recruits bone marrow-derived fibroblast precursors in renal fibrosis. *J. Am. Soc. Nephrol.* **2011**, *22*, 1876–1886. [CrossRef] [PubMed]

34. Anscher, M.S.; Kong, F.M.; Andrews, K.; Clough, R.; Marks, L.B.; Bentel, G.; Jirtle, R.L. Plasma transforming growth factor beta1 as a predictor of radiation pneumonitis. *Int. J. Radiat. Oncol. Biol. Phys.* **1998**, *41*, 1029–1035. [CrossRef]

35. Mazeron, R.; Etienne-Mastroianni, B.; Perol, D.; Arpin, D.; Vincent, M.; Falchero, L.; Martel-Lafay, I.; Carrie, C.; Claude, L. Predictive factors of late radiation fibrosis: A prospective study in non-small cell lung cancer. *Int. J. Radiat. Oncol. Biol. Phys.* **2010**, *77*, 38–43. [CrossRef] [PubMed]

36. Chen, Y.; Rubin, P.; Williams, J.; Hernady, E.; Smudzin, T.; Okunieff, P. Circulating IL-6 as a predictor of radiation pneumonitis. *Int. J. Radiat. Oncol. Biol. Phys.* **2001**, *49*, 641–648. [CrossRef]

37. Selman, M.; Ruiz, V.; Cabrera, S.; Segura, L.; Ramirez, R.; Barrios, R.; Pardo, A. TIMP-1, -2, -3, and -4 in idiopathic pulmonary fibrosis. A prevailing nondegradative lung microenvironment? *Am. J. Physiol. Lung Cell Mol. Physiol.* **2000**, *279*, L562–L574. [CrossRef] [PubMed]

38. Ruiz, V.; Ordonez, R.M.; Berumen, J.; Ramirez, R.; Uhal, B.; Becerril, C.; Pardo, A.; Selman, M. Unbalanced collagenases/TIMP-1 expression and epithelial apoptosis in experimental lung fibrosis. *Am. J. Physiol. Lung Cell Mol. Physiol.* **2003**, *285*, L1026–L1036. [CrossRef] [PubMed]

39. Wynn, T.A. Integrating mechanisms of pulmonary fibrosis. *J. Exp. Med.* **2011**, *208*, 1339–1350. [CrossRef] [PubMed]

40. Li, D.; Guabiraba, R.; Besnard, A.G.; Komai-Koma, M.; Jabir, M.S.; Zhang, L.; Graham, G.J.; Kurowska-Stolarska, M.; Liew, F.Y.; McSharry, C.; et al. IL-33 promotes ST2-dependent lung fibrosis by the induction of alternatively activated macrophages and innate lymphoid cells in mice. *J. Allergy Clin. Immunol.* **2014**, *134*, 1422–1432. [CrossRef] [PubMed]

41. Hasegawa, M.; Sato, S.; Takehara, K. Augmented production of chemokines (monocyte chemotactic protein-1 (MCP-1), macrophage inflammatory protein-1alpha (MIP-1alpha) and (MIP-1beta) in patients with systemic sclerosis: MCP-1 and MIP-1alpha may be involved in the development of pulmonary fibrosis. *Clin. Exp. Immunol.* **1999**, *117*, 159–165. [PubMed]

42. Car, B.D.; Meloni, F.; Luisetti, M.; Semenzato, G.; Gialdroni-Grassi, G.; Walz, A. Elevated IL-8 and MCP-1 in the bronchoalveolar lavage fluid of patients with idiopathic pulmonary fibrosis and pulmonary sarcoidosis. *Am. J. Respir. Crit. Care Med.* **1994**, *149*, 655–659. [CrossRef] [PubMed]

43. Piguet, P.F.; Vesin, C.; Grau, G.E.; Thompson, R.C. Interleukin 1 receptor antagonist (IL-1ra) prevents or cures pulmonary fibrosis elicited in mice by bleomycin or silica. *Cytokine* **1993**, *5*, 57–61. [CrossRef]

44. Mall, M.; Grubb, B.R.; Harkema, J.R.; O'Neal, W.K.; Boucher, R.C. Increased airway epithelial Na$^+$ absorption produces cystic fibrosis-like lung disease in mice. *Nat. Med.* **2004**, *10*, 487–493. [CrossRef] [PubMed]

45. Hagiwara, S.I.; Ishii, Y.; Kitamura, S. Aerosolized administration of N-acetylcysteine attenuates lung fibrosis induced by bleomycin in mice. *Am. J. Respir. Crit. Care Med.* **2000**, *162*, 225–231. [CrossRef] [PubMed]

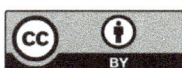

marine drugs

MDPI

Article

Components from the Leaves and Twigs of Mangrove *Lumnitzera racemosa* with Anti-Angiogenic and Anti-Inflammatory Effects

Szu-Yin Yu [1,†], Shih-Wei Wang [1,2,†], Tsong-Long Hwang [3,4,5], Bai-Luh Wei [6], Chien-Jung Su [1], Fang-Rong Chang [1,7,*] and Yuan-Bin Cheng [1,8,*]

[1] Graduate Institute of Natural Products, College of Pharmacy, Kaohsiung Medical University, Kaohsiung 807, Taiwan; s91412232@gmail.com (S.-Y.Y.); shihwei@mmc.edu.tw (S.-W.W.); scj820826@gmail.com (C.-J.S.)

[2] Department of Medicine, Mackay Medical College, New Taipei City 252, Taiwan

[3] Graduate Institute of Natural Products, College of Medicine, and Chinese Herbal Medicine Research Team, Healthy Aging Research Center, Chang Gung University, Taoyuan 333, Taiwan; htl@mail.cgu.edu.tw

[4] Research Center for Chinese Herbal Medicine, Research Center for Food and Cosmetic Safety, and Graduate Institute of Health Industry Technology, College of Human Ecology, Chang Gung University of Science and Technology, Taoyuan 333, Taiwan

[5] Department of Anesthesiology, Chang Gung Memorial Hospital, Taoyuan 333, Taiwan

[6] Department of Life Science, National Taitung University, Taitung 950, Taiwan; blwei@nttu.edu.tw

[7] National Research Institute of Chinese Medicine, Ministry of Health and Welfare, Taipei 112, Taiwan

[8] Department of Medical Research, Kaohsiung Medical University Hospital, Kaohsiung 807, Taiwan

*   Correspondence: aaronfrc@kmu.edu.tw (F.-R.C.); jmb@kmu.edu.tw (Y.-B.C.); Tel.: +886-7-312-1101 (ext. 2162) (F.-R.C.); +886-7-312-1101 (ext. 2197) (Y.-B.C.)

† These authors contributed equally to this work.

Received: 5 October 2018; Accepted: 23 October 2018; Published: 25 October 2018

Abstract: One new neolignan, racelactone A (**1**), together with seven known compounds (**2**−**8**) were isolated from the methanolic extract of the leaves and twigs of *Lumnitzera racemosa*. The structure of racelactone A (**1**) was determined on the basis of the mass and NMR spectroscopic data interpretation. With respect to bioactivity, compound 1 displayed an anti-angiogenic effect by suppressing tube formation. Furthermore, compounds **1**, **4**, and **5** showed significant anti-inflammatory effects with IC_{50} values of 4.95 ± 0.89, 1.95 ± 0.40, and 2.57 ± 0.23 μM, respectively. The plausible biosynthesis pathway of racelactone A (**1**) was proposed.

Keywords: neolignan; *Lumnitzera racemosa*; anti-angiogenesis; anti-inflammation

1. Introduction

Mangroves are unique plants growing in the intertidal zone of the tropical and subtropical climates; these species are salt-tolerant and have mechanisms which affect a variety of cellular metabolic processes [1]. Plants of the mangrove genus *Lumnitzera* (Combretaceae) comprise more than 600 species in Asia, Austria, and Africa. Among them, *Lumnitzera racemosa* Willd. is native to the seashore of southern Taiwan. *L. racemosa* can grow up to a five-meter height; its bark is dark brown and rough, the leaves are slightly concave top round, and the fruits are drupe and with an ellipsoid shape [2]. The woods of *L. racemosa* are hard and have a long shelf life; they can be used as building materials, equipment, or fuels. *L. racemosa* is also fantabulous nectar plant, while the leaves are edible to date [3]. Traditionally, the sap of this plant is used to treat cutaneous pruritus, herpes, scabies, and thrush [4]. The chemical constituents of *L. racemosa* are fatty acids, flavonoids, polyisoprenoid alcohols, tannins, and triterpenoids [5]. Pharmacological studies of the extracts from *L. racemosa* demonstrated antibacterial, antifungal, antihypertensive, antioxidant, cytotoxic, and hepatoprotective activities [6–9].

Inflammation is tightly associated with carcinogenesis and the disease progression of cancer [10]. Angiogenesis has been reported to facilitate the growth and dissemination of cancer cells in tumor microenvironments [11]. Plentiful studies reveal that inhibition of inflammation and angiogenesis is an effective therapeutic strategy to suppress cancer development and metastasis [12,13]. Our preliminary pharmacological investigation indicated that methanolic extract of the leaves and twigs of *L. racemosa* exerted promising anti-angiogenic and anti-inflammatory responses. Herein, we describe the isolation, structural elucidation, and bioactivities of one new neolignan, racelactone A (**1**), along with seven known compounds (**2–8**).

2. Results

In the present study, the methanolic extracted from *L. racemosa* was partitioned with ethyl acetate (EtOAc) and water (H_2O). The EtOAc layer was further partitioned with *n*-hexane and 75% methanol (MeOH) in H_2O to give a 75% $MeOH_{(aq)}$ layer. One new compound, racelactone A (**1**), and seven known compounds: Botulin (**2**) [14,15], 3,4,3'-tri-*O*-methyl ellagic acid (**3**) [16], methyl gallate (**4**) [17], myricitrin (**5**) [18], stigmasterol (**6**) [19], kaempferol (**7**) [20], and isoguaiacin (**8**) [21] were identified from the 75% $MeOH_{(aq)}$ layer. The structures of compounds (**1–8**) are shown in Figure 1.

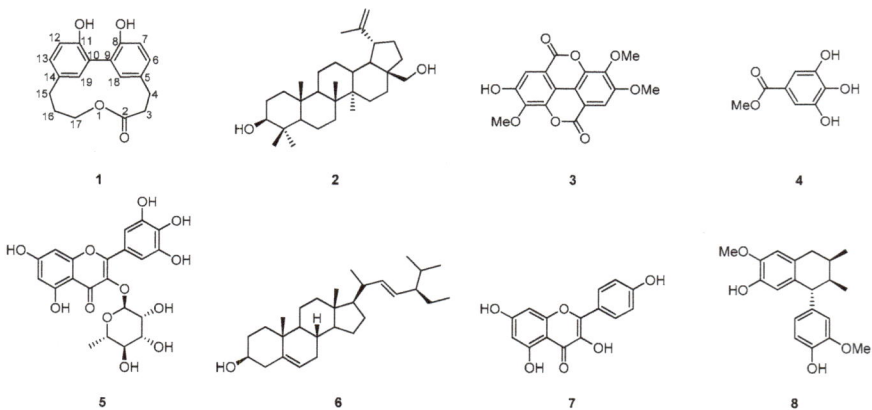

Figure 1. Structures of compounds **1−8**.

Racelactone A (**1**) was isolated as an amorphous powder, light yellow, having a molecular formula determined as $C_{18}H_{18}O_4$. Ten indices of hydrogen deficiency were calculated, in accord with the high-resolution electrospray ionisation mass spectrometry (HRESIMS) data (*m*/*z* 321.10955 [M + Na]$^+$) (Figure S1) and NMR spectrum. The IR spectrum (Figure S2) of **1** suggested the presence of hydroxy (3364 cm^{-1}), carbonyl (1709 cm^{-1}) and aromatic (1503, 1586 cm^{-1}) functionalities. In ^{1}H NMR (Figure S3), data revealed six olefinic methines (δ_H 6.81, 6.87, 7.01, 7.03, 7.06, and 7.18), and five methylenes (δ_H 2.25, 2.58, 2.82, 2.98, and 4.29) (Table 1). The ^{13}C (Figure S4) and DEPT NMR spectrum (Table 1) of **1** noted eighteen carbon signals, including one carbonyl (δc 175.0), six olefinic methines (δc 113.3, 115.9, 116.4, 128.3, 129.2, and 133.1), six nonprotonated carbons (δc 126.6, 127.2, 131.4, 132.7, 151.9, and 152.7), and five methylenes (δc 25.2, 29.7, 30.7, 35.7, and 65.7). Analyses on a set of signals and coupling constants at δ_H 6.87 (d, 1H, *J* = 8.2 Hz, H-12), 7.03 (dd, 1H, *J* = 8.2, 2.4 Hz, H-13), and 7.06 (d, 1H, *J* = 2.5 Hz, H-18) as well as another set at δ_H 7.01 (dd, 1H, *J* = 8.2, 2.5 Hz, H-6), 6.81 (d, 1H, *J* = 8.1 Hz, H-7), and 7.19 (d, 1H, *J* = 2.5 Hz, H-19) led to the identification of two 1,3,4-trisubstituted phenyl moieties. From analyses of the NMR, UV (Figure S5), and IR data, compound **1** was determined to be a neolignan. Compound **1** showed similar ^{1}H and ^{13}C NMR signals (Table 1), partially similar to those of corniculatolide A, which has an ether bridge between two propylphenyl moieties [22,23]—except for the presence of two unusual quaternary carbon signals at δc 126.6 and δc 127.2 instead of two signals at δc 149.0 and δc 154.2 in corniculatolide A. This indicated a new carbon–carbon linkage formation in the target molecule.

Table 1. ^{1}H and ^{13}C NMR data of $\mathbf{1}^a$ in acetone-d_6.

Position	δ_H, mult (*J* in Hz)	δ_C, Type	HMBC (^{1}H-^{13}C)
2	-	175.0, C	-
3	2.58, m	35.7, CH$_2$	2, 4, 5
4	2.98, m	29.7, CH$_2$	2, 3, 5, 6, 18
5	-	132.7, C	-
6	7.01, dd (8.1, 2.5)	128.3, CH	7, 8, 18
7	6.81, d (8.1)	115.9, CH	5, 6, 8, 9
8	-	152.7, C	-
9	-	127.2, C	-
10	-	126.6, C	-
11	-	151.9, C	-
12	6.87, d (8.2)	116.4, CH	10, 11, 14
13	7.03, dd (8.2, 2.5)	129.2, CH	11, 12, 15, 19
14	-	131.4, C	-
15	2.82, m	30.7, CH$_2$	13, 14, 16, 17, 19
16	2.25, m	25.2, CH$_2$	14, 15, 17
17	4.29, t (5.0)	65.7, CH$_2$	2, 15, 16
18	7.06, d (2.5)	133.1, CH	4, 6, 8, 10
19	7.19, d (2.5)	133.3, CH	9, 11, 13

^{a} ^{1}H and ^{13}C NMR data (δ) were measured at 400 and 100 MHz, respectively; chemical shifts are in ppm.

The planar structure of **1** was established by the correlation spectroscopy (COSY) (Figure S6) and heter onuclear multiple bond correlation (HMBC) (Figure S7) correlations (Figure 2). The COSY correlations established the fragments of H-3/H-4, H-6/H-7, H-12/H-13, and H-15/H-16/H-17 of compound **1**. The HMBC correlations of H-4/C-5, C-6, and C-18 and the correlations of H-15/C-13, C-14, and C-19 determined the linkages of two sets of propyl and phenyl functions, respectively. The macroring connection system of two phenylpropanoid moieties was completed on the basis of a key HMBC correlation between H-17/C-2, H-18/C-10, and H-19/C-9. As mentioned above, compound **1** was categorized as a macrolactone, and named racelactone A. The biosynthesis of racelactone A is proposed to be initiated by a PAL enzyme of phenylalanine to form dihydrocaffeic acid. The precursor was resonated to form intermediates A and B. Phenoxy radicals of intermediates A and B were linked to generate the intermediate C, which was structured as racelactone A during a cyclization (Figure 3).

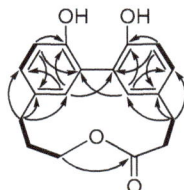

Figure 2. COSY (bold bond) and selected HMBC (arrow) correlations of **1**.

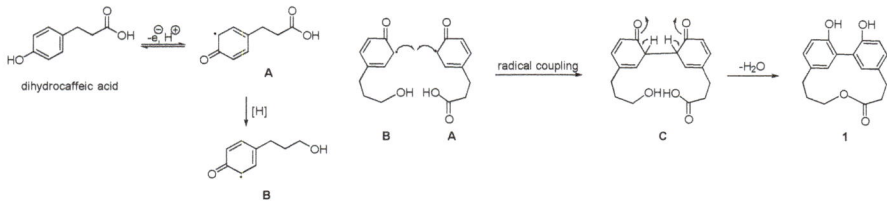

Figure 3. Plausible biosynthesis pathway of racelactone A (**1**).

Circulating endothelial progenitor cells (EPCs) have been reported to promote tumor angiogenesis and metastasis [24,25]. Tumors can secrete a variety of angiogenic factors to induce the recruitment of EPCs from bone marrow to the tumor site. Recruited EPCs enter the circulation system from their niche in bone marrow and extravasate with the chemotactic stimuli. After reaching the tumor site, EPCs differentiate into the structural part of the tumor vasculature, which contributes to tumor progression. Furthermore, EPCs have the ability to release pro-inflammatory cytokines that facilitate the growth and metastatic spread of tumors. Compelling evidence suggests that selective targeting of EPCs represents a novel therapeutic strategy for cancer treatment [26]. The differentiation and formation of capillary vessels is the most critical process during EPCs angiogenesis. Therefore, we performed tube formation assay to evaluate the anti-angiogenic activity of racelactone A in EPCs. As shown in Figure 4, the capillary tube-like structure was suppressed by racelactone A in a concentration-dependent manner. Sorafenib, a well-known angiogenesis inhibitor, was used as the positive control. To confirm this anti-angiogenic effect was not caused by the potential cytotoxicity of racelactone A, the release of lactate dehydrogenase (LDH) was measured in racelactone A-treated EPCs. We found that no statistical difference was observed between the control EPCs and EPCs treated with racelactone A. Collectively, these results reveal that the anti-angiogenic effect of racelactone A is not due to the cytotoxic action in human EPCs.

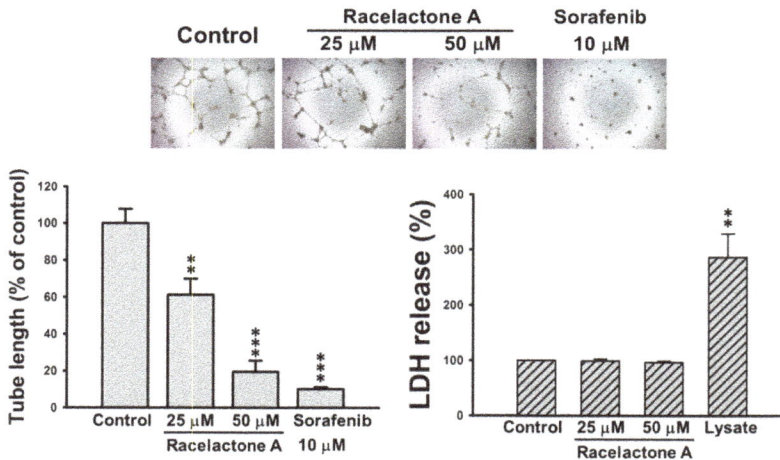

Figure 4. Effect of racelactone A (**1**) on tube formation and cytotoxicity of human endothelial progenitor cells (EPCs). EPCs were with the indicated concentrations of racelactone A and sorafenib for 24 h. The capillary-like structure formation and lactate dehydrogenase (LDH) release were determined by tube formation and cytotoxicity assay, respectively. Representative images of EPCs' tube formation were shown (phase contrast, 40×). Data represent the mean ± SEM of five independent experiments. ** $p < 0.01$, *** $p < 0.001$ compared with the control group.

All compounds were subjected to anti-inflammatory assays on superoxide anion generation and elastase release in fMLF/CB-induced human neutrophils inhibitory effects. Fortunately, the new compound **1** selectively displayed significant inhibitory activity on superoxide anion generation ($IC_{50} = 4.95 \pm 0.89$ µM). The known compounds **4** and **5** also showed strong activity (Table 2).

Table 2. Inhibitory effects of isolates on superoxide anion generation and elastase release in fMLF/CB-induced human neutrophils.

Compound	Percentage of IC_{50} (µM) [a]			
	Superoxide Anion		Elastase Release	
1	4.95 ± 0.89	**	>10	
4	1.95 ± 0.40	***	>10	
5	2.57 ± 0.23	***	>10	
genistein [b]	1.54 ± 0.37	***	17.47 ± 2.80	***

Percentage of inhibition (Inh %) at 10 µM concentration. Results are presented as mean $\pm$ SEM (n = 3~5). ** $p < 0.01$, *** $p < 0.001$ compared with the control. [a] Concentration necessary for 50% inhibition (IC_{50}). [b] positive control.

3. Materials and Methods

3.1. General Experimental Procedures

Optical rotation was measured on a JASCO P-1020 digital polarimeter (Tokyo, Japan). UV data were recorded on a JASCO V-530 UV/VIS Spectrophotometer (Tokyo, Japan). High-resolution ESIMS data were obtained on a Bruker APEX II spectrometer (Billerica, MA, USA)). The IR spectrum was measured on a Perkin Elmer system 2000 FT-IR spectrophotometer (Waltham, MA, USA). The NMR spectra were obtained by JEOL JNM-ECS 400 MHz NMR (Akishima, Japan). Merck (Darmstadt, Germany) silica gel 60 and GE Healthcare (Chicago, IL, USA) Sephadex LH-20 were used for column chromatography. The instrumentation for HPLC was composed of a Shimadzu LC-10AD pump (Kyoto, Japan) and a Shimadzu SPD-M10A PDA detector.

3.2. Material

Specimens of *Lumnitzera racemosa* were collected in south Taiwan, in August 2015. The research samples were identified by Yuan-Bin Cheng. A voucher specimen (no. KMU-LR01) was deposited in the Graduate Institute of Natural Products, College of Pharmacy, Kaohsiung Medical University.

3.3. Extraction and Isolation

The air-dry twigs and leaves (15.0 kg) of *L. racemosa* were ground and extracted thrice with MeOH (40 L) at room temperature. The solvent was concentrated under reducing pressure to yield crude extracts. The MeOH crude extracts were partitioned between H_2O/EtOAc (1:1) to afford two portions. The EtOAc part was partitioned with *n*-hexane and 75% MeOH in water (1:1). The 75% $MeOH_{(aq)}$ layer (88.5 g) was subjected to a silica gel column stepwise eluted with *n*-hexane/EtOAc to yield botulin (221.1 mg), 3,4,3′-Tri-*O*-methyl ellagic acid (3330.0 mg), methyl gallate (4730.0 mg), myricitrin (5599.5 mg), and six fractions (A−J). Fraction C (830 mg) was isolated by silica gel column to give stigmasterol (63.4 mg). Fraction E (2.4 g) was chromatographed over a silica gel column to afford six subfractions (E.1−E.6). Subfraction E.4 (196.9 mg) was further separated by an LH-20 column, eluted with 100% MeOH to yield kaempferol (712.8 mg). Racelactone A (111.0 mg) and isoguaiacin (83.7 mg) were obtained from subfraction D.1 (144.7 mg) by LH-20 column, eluted with 100% MeOH and Phenyl-hexyl column (Luna phenyl-hexyl, 100 Å, 250 × 10 mm, Phenomenex®) stepwise from 70% to 100% $MeOH_{(aq)}$.

Racelactone A (1): Light yellow amorphous powder; $[\alpha]_D^{26}$ -0.6 (*c* 0.05, MeOH); UV (MeOH) λ_{max} (log ε) 299 (2.85), 252 (2.95), 215 (3.34) nm; IR (neat) v_{max}: 3364, 1709, 1503, 1411 cm^{-1}; ^{1}H NMR and ^{13}C NMR data, see Table 1; HRESIMS *m/z* 321.10955 [M + Na]$^+$ (calcd for $C_{18}H_{18}O_4Na^+$: 321.10973).

3.4. Preparation of Human EPCs

The ethical approval for the collection of human EPCs was granted by the Institutional Review Board of Mackay Medical College, New Taipei City, Taiwan (P1000002). Prior to collecting the peripheral blood from healthy donors, informed consent was acquired. After density centrifugation Ficoll-Paque plus (Amersham Biosciences, Uppala, Sweden), peripheral blood mononuclear cells (PBMCs) were isolated from the fractionated blood components. CD34-positive progenitor cells were isolated from PMBCs with CD34 MicroBead kit and MACS Cell Separation System (Miltenyi Biotec, Bergisch Gladbach, Germany). Further isolation and preservation of CD34-positive EPCs were performed as described previously [27,28]. In the present study, all experiments were carried out on EPCs between passages 10 and 18. EPCs were cultured with 1% gelatin-coated plasticware and MV2 complete medium (PromoCell, Heidelberg, Germany) with 20% defined fetal bovine serum (FBS) (HyClone, Logan, UT, USA) in humidified incubator containing 5% CO_2 at 37 °C.

3.5. Tube Formation Assay

The capillary tube formation assay was carried out on Matrigel-coated 96-well plates. EPCs were seeded with the density of 1.25×10^4 cells per well and incubated in an MV2 complete medium with 2% FBS and the indicated concentration of tested compounds for 24 h at 37 °C. Quantifications of EPCs differentiation and capillary-like tube formation were done with photomicrographs taken by an inverted phase contrast microscope. The long axis of each tube was measured with Image J software in 3 randomly chosen fields per well.

3.6. Cytotoxicity Assay

5×10^3 of EPCs per well were seeded onto 96-well plates and incubated with an MV2 complete medium containing 2% FBS in the presence of vehicle (DMSO) or racelactone A. The quantification of LDH release in the medium was done with a cytotoxicity assay kit (Promega, Madison, WI, USA).

3.7. Superoxide Anion and Elastase Release Assays

The assay on superoxide anion generation and elastase release in response to fMLF stimulation of neutrophils were assayed by the same method as those of the reference published by co-author Professor Tsong-Long Hwang [29].

4. Conclusions

In summary, eight compounds, including one unusual macrolactone neolignan, were isolated and identified during a phytochemical investigation of the Taiwanese mangrove, *L. racemosa*. The new compound shows promising activities to anti-angiogenic and anti-inflammatory effects. Our findings suggest that racelactone A (**1**) may serve as a lead compound worthy of further development against angiogenesis-related diseases or inflammation-facilitated disorders, especially for the treatment of cancer.

Supplementary Materials: The following are available online at http://www.mdpi.com/1660-3397/16/11/404/s1, Figure S1: HRESIMS of racelactone A (**1**). Figure S2: IR spectrum of racelactone A (**1**). Figure S3: ^{1}H NMR Spectrum of racelactone A (**1**) in acetone-d_6. Figure S4: ^{13}C NMR Spectrum of racelactone A (**1**) in acetone-d_6. Figure S5: UV spectrum of racelactone A (**1**). Figure S6: COSY Spectrum of racelactone A (**1**) in acetone-d_6. Figure S7: HMBC Spectrum of racelactone A (**1**) in acetone-d_6.

Author Contributions: S.-Y.Y., S.-W.W., B.-L.W., F.-R.C., and Y.-B.C. contributed to manuscript preparation; Y.-B.C. designed the whole experiment; S.-W.W., T.-L.H., and C.-J.S. analyzed the data and performed data acquisition.

Funding: This research was funded by [Ministry of Science and Technology, Taiwan] grant number [MOST 105-2628-B-037-001-MY3, MOST 106-2320-B-037-008-MY2, MOST106-2320-B-037-016, and MOST 107-2628-B-037-001].

Acknowledgments: We appreciated the Ministry of Science and Technology, Taiwan (MOST 105-2628-B-037-001-MY3 and MOST 106-2320-B-037-008-MY2 award to F.-R. Chang; MOST106-2320-B-037-016 and MOST 107-2628-B-037-001 award to Y.-B. Cheng).

Conflicts of Interest: The authors declare no conflict of interest.

References

1. Parida, A.L.; Jha, B. Salt tolerance mechanisms in mangroves: A review. *Trees* **2010**, *24*, 199–217. [CrossRef]
2. Chen, J. *Flora of China*; Missouri Botanical Garden: St. Louis, MO, USA; Harvard University Herbaria: Cambridge, MA, USA, 2007; Volume 13, p. 310.
3. Tomlinson, P.B. *The Botany of Mangroves*; Cambridge University Press: Cambridge, UK, 2016; p. 236, ISBN 9781107080676.
4. Chong, K.Y.; Tan, H.T.W.; Corlett, R.T. *A Checklist of the Total Vascular Plant Flora of Singapore Native, Naturalized and Cultivated Species*; National University of Singapore: Singapore, 2009; p. 273.
5. Anjaneyulu, A.S.R.; Murthy, Y.L.N.; Rao, V.L.; Sreedhar, K. A new aromatic ester from the mangrove plant *Lumnitzera racemosa* willd[+]. *ARKIVOC* **2003**, *3*, 25–30. [CrossRef]
6. Lin, T.C.; Hsu, F.L.; Cheng, J.T. Antihypertensive activity of corilagin and chebulinic acid, tannins from *Lumnitzera racemosa*. *J. Nat. Prod.* **1993**, *56*, 629–632. [CrossRef]
7. D'Souza, L.; Wahidulla, S.; Devi, P. Antibacterial phenolics from the mangrove *Lumnitzera racemosa*. *Indian J. Mar. Sci.* **2010**, *39*, 294–298.
8. Ravikumar, S.; Gnanadesigan, M. Hepatoprotective and antioxidant activity of a mangrove plant *Lumnitzera racemosa*. *Asian Pac. J. Trop. Biomed.* **2011**, *1*, 348–352. [CrossRef]
9. Thao, N.P.; Luyen, B.T.T.; Diep, C.N.; Tai, B.H.; Kim, E.J.; Kang, H.K.; Lee, S.H.; Jang, H.D.; Cuong, N.T.; Thanh, N.V.; et al. In vitro evaluation of the antioxidant and cytotoxic activities of constituents of the mangrove *Lumnitzera racemosa* Willd. *Arch. Pharm. Res.* **2015**, *38*, 446–455. [CrossRef] [PubMed]
10. Clevers, H. At the crossroads of inflammation and cancer. *Cell* **2004**, *118*, 671–674. [CrossRef] [PubMed]
11. Chung, A.S.; Lee, J.; Ferrara, N. Targeting the tumour vasculature: Insights from physiological angiogenesis. *Nat. Rev. Cancer* **2010**, *10*, 505–514. [CrossRef] [PubMed]
12. Weis, S.M.; Cheresh, D.A. Tumor angiogenesis: Molecular pathways and therapeutic targets. *Nat. Med.* **2011**, *17*, 1359–1370. [CrossRef] [PubMed]
13. Zha, S.; Yegnasubramanian, V.; Nelson, W.G.; Isaacs, W.B.; Marzo, A.M.D. Cyclooxygenases in cancer: Progress and perspective. *Cancer Lett.* **2004**, *215*, 1–20. [CrossRef] [PubMed]
14. Liao, C.-R.; Kuo, Y.-H.; Ho, Y.-L.; Wang, C.-Y.; Yang, C.-S.; Lin, C.-W.; Chang, Y.-S. Studies on cytotoxic constituents from the leaves of *Elaeagnus oldhamii* Maxim. in non-small cell lung cancer A549 Cells. *Molecules* **2014**, *19*, 9515–9534. [CrossRef] [PubMed]
15. Schmidt, J.; Himmelreich, U.; Adam, G. Brassinosteroids, sterols and lup-20(29)-en-2α,3β,28-triol from *Rheum Rhabarbarum*. *Phytochemistry* **1995**, *40*, 527–531. [CrossRef]
16. Begum, S.S.; Tauseef, S.; Siddiqui, B.S.; Nizami, S.S.; Ghulam, H.; Ahmad, A. In vitro antibacterial and antifungal activity of flower buds (clove) of *Syzygium aromaticum*. *J. Chem. Soc. Pak.* **2014**, *36*, 723–728.
17. Madikizela, B.; Aderogba, M.A.; Finnie, J.F.; Staden, J.V. Isolation and characterization of antimicrobial compounds from *Terminalia phanerophlebia* Engl. & Diels leaf extracts. *J. Ethnopharmacol.* **2014**, *156*, 228–234. [CrossRef] [PubMed]
18. Saldanha, L.L.; Vilegas, W.; Dokkedal, A.L. Characterization of flavonoids and phenolic acids in *Myrcia bella* Cambess. using FIA-ESI-IT-MS[n] and HPLC-PAD-ESI-IT-MS combined with NMR. *Molecules* **2013**, *18*, 8402–8416. [CrossRef] [PubMed]
19. Forgo, P.; Kövér, K.E. Gradient enhanced selective experiments in the ^{1}H NMR chemical shift assignment of the skeleton and side-chain resonances of stigmasterol, a phytosterol derivative. *Steroids* **2004**, *69*, 43–50. [CrossRef] [PubMed]
20. Moraes, L.S.; Donza, M.R.H.; Rodrigues, A.P.D.; Silva, B.J.M.; Brasil, A.S.B.; Zoghbi, M.G.B.; Andrade, E.H.A.; Guilhon, G.M.S.P.; Silva, E.O. Leishmanicidal activity of (+)-phyllanthidine and the phytochemical profile of *Margaritaria nobilis* (Phyllanthaceae). *Molecules* **2015**, *20*, 22157–22169. [CrossRef] [PubMed]

21. Wang, B.-G.; Hong, X.; Li, L.; Zhou, J.; Hao, Z.-J. Chemical constituents of two Chinese Magnoliaceae plants, *Tsoongiodendron odorum* and *Manglietiastrum sinicum*, and their inhibition of platelet aggregation. *Planta Med.* **2000**, *66*, 511–515. [CrossRef] [PubMed]

22. Vongvanich, N.; Kittakoop, P.; Charoenchai, P.; Intamas, S.; Danwisetkanjana, K.; Thebtaranonth, Y. Combretastatins D-3 and D-4, new macrocyclic lactones from *Getonia floribunda*. *Planta Med.* **2005**, *71*, 191–193. [CrossRef] [PubMed]

23. Pettit, G.R.; Quistorf, P.D.; Fry, J.A.; Herald, D.L.; Hamel, E.; Chapuis, J.-C. Antineoplastic agents. 565. synthesis of combretastatin D-2 phosphate and dihydro-combretastatin D-2[1]. *J. Nat. Prod.* **2009**, *72*, 876–883. [CrossRef] [PubMed]

24. Carmeliet, P. Angiogenesis in life, disease and medicine. *Nature* **2005**, *438*, 932–936. [CrossRef] [PubMed]

25. Urbich, C.; Dimmeler, S. Endothelial progenitor cells: Characterization and role in vascular biology. *Circ. Res.* **2004**, *95*, 343–353. [CrossRef] [PubMed]

26. Moschetta, M.; Mishima, Y.; Sahin, I.; Manier, S.; Glavey, S.; Vacca, A.; Roccaro, A.M.; Ghobrial, I.M. Role of endothelial progenitor cells in cancer progression. *BBA-Rev. Cancer* **2014**, *1846*, 26–39. [CrossRef] [PubMed]

27. Chung, C.-H.; Chang, C.-H.; Chen, S.-S.; Wang, H.-H.; Yen, J.-Y.; Hsiao, C.-J.; Wu, N.-L.; Chen, Y.-L.; Huang, T.-F.; Wang, P.-C.; et al. Butein inhibits angiogenesis of human endothelial progenitor cells via the translation dependent signaling pathway. *Evid.-Based Complement. Altern. Med.* **2013**, *2013*, e943187. [CrossRef] [PubMed]

28. Lee, M.-S.; Wang, S.-W.; Wang, G.-J.; Pang, K.-L.; Lee, C.-K.; Kuo, Y.-H.; Cha, H.-J.; Lin, R.-K.; Lee, T.-H. Angiogenesis inhibitors and anti-inflammatory agents from *Phoma* sp. NTOU4195. *J. Nat. Prod.* **2016**, *79*, 2983–2990. [CrossRef] [PubMed]

29. Yang, S.-C.; Chung, P.-J.; Ho, C.-M.; Kuo, C.-Y.; Hung, M.-F.; Huang, Y.-T.; Chang, W.-Y.; Chang, Y.-W.; Chan, K.-H.; Hwang, T.-L. Propofol inhibits superoxide production, elastase release, and chemotaxis in formyl peptide–activated human neutrophils by blocking formyl peptide receptor 1. *J. Immunol.* **2013**, *190*, 6511–6519. [CrossRef] [PubMed]

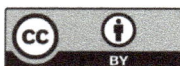

marine drugs

MDPI

Article

Phomaketide A Inhibits Lymphangiogenesis in Human Lymphatic Endothelial Cells

Huai-Ching Tai [1,2,†], Tzong-Huei Lee [3], Chih-Hsin Tang [4,5,6], Lei-Po Chen [7,8,†], Wei-Cheng Chen [7,8], Ming-Shian Lee [3], Pei-Chi Chen [9], Chih-Yang Lin [9], Chih-Wen Chi [10], Yu-Jen Chen [10,11], Cheng-Ta Lai [12], Shiou-Sheng Chen [13,14], Kuang-Wen Liao [8,15,16], Chien-Hsing Lee [17,18,*] and Shih-Wei Wang [9,19,*]

[1] School of Medicine, Fu-Jen Catholic University, New Taipei City 242, Taiwan; taihuai48@hotmail.com
[2] Department of Urology, Fu-Jen Catholic University Hospital, New Taipei City 242, Taiwan
[3] Institute of Fisheries Science, National Taiwan University, Taipei 106, Taiwan; thlee1@ntu.edu.tw (T.-H.L.); d301101010@tmu.edu.tw (M.-S.L.)
[4] Chinese Medicine Research Center, China Medical University, Taichung 404, Taiwan; chtang@mail.cmu.edu.tw
[5] Department of Pharmacology, School of Medicine, China Medical University, Taichung 404, Taiwan
[6] Department of Biotechnology, College of Health Science, Asia University, Taichung 413, Taiwan
[7] Department of Orthopaedics, MacKay Memorial Hospital, Taipei 104, Taiwan; robert82ccc@gmail.com (L.-P.C.); wchena7648@gmail.com (W.-C.C.)
[8] Ph.D. Degree Program of Biomedical Science and Engineering, National Chiao Tung University, Hsinchu 300, Taiwan; liaonms@pchome.com.tw
[9] Department of Medicine, Mackay Medical College, New Taipei City 252, Taiwan; 1622689043new@gmail.com (P.-C.C.); p123400@hotmail.com (C.-Y.L.)
[10] Department of Medical Research, MacKay Memorial Hospital, New Taipei City 251, Taiwan; d48906003@yahoo.com.tw (C.-W.C.); chenmdphd@gmail.com (Y.-J.C.)
[11] Department of Radiation Oncology, MacKay Memorial Hospital, Taipei 104, Taiwan
[12] Division of Colon and Rectal Surgery, Department of Surgery, MacKay Memorial Hospital, Taipei 104, Taiwan; laichengta@gmail.com
[13] Division of Urology, Taipei City Hospital HepingFuyou Branch, Taipei 100, Taiwan; DAB67@tpech.gov.tw
[14] Commission for General Education, National United University, Miaoli 360, Taiwan
[15] Institute of Molecular Medicine and Bioengineering, National Chiao Tung University, Hsinchu 300, Taiwan
[16] Department of Biotechnology and Bioindustry Sciences, National Cheng Kung University, Tainan 300, Taiwan
[17] Department of Pharmacology, Graduate Institute of Medicine, College of Medicine, Kaohsiung Medical University, Kaohsiung 807, Taiwan
[18] Department of Medical Research, Kaohsiung Medical University Hospital, Kaohsiung 807, Taiwan
[19] Graduate Institute of Natural Products, College of Pharmacy, Kaohsiung Medical University, Kaohsiung 807, Taiwan
*   Correspondence: chlee0818@gmail.com (C.-H.L.); shihwei@mmc.edu.tw (S.-W.W.); Tel.: +886-7-312-1101 #2139-14 (C.-H.L.); +886-2-26360303 #1219 (S.-W.W.)
† These authors contributed equally to this work.

Received: 27 February 2019; Accepted: 2 April 2019; Published: 6 April 2019

Abstract: Lymphangiogenesis is an important biological process associated with cancer metastasis. The development of new drugs that block lymphangiogenesis represents a promising therapeutic strategy. Marine fungus-derived compound phomaketide A, isolated from the fermented broth of *Phoma* sp. NTOU4195, has been reported to exhibit anti-angiogenic and anti-inflammatory effects. However, its anti-lymphangiogenic activity has not been clarified to date. In this study, we showed that phomaketide A inhibited cell growth, migration, and tube formation of lymphatic endothelial cells (LECs) without an evidence of cytotoxicity. Mechanistic investigations revealed that phomaketide A reduced LECs-induced lymphangiogenesis via vascular endothelial growth factor receptor-3 (VEGFR-3), protein kinase Cδ (PKCδ), and endothelial nitric oxide synthase (eNOS) signalings. Furthermore, human proteome array analysis indicated that phomaketide A significantly enhanced the protein levels of various protease inhibitors, including cystatin A, serpin B6, tissue factor pathway inhibitor (TFPI), and tissue inhibitor matrix metalloproteinase 1 (TIMP-1). Importantly, phomaketide A impeded tumor growth and lymphangiogenesis by decreasing the expression of LYVE-1, a specific marker for lymphatic vessels, in tumor xenograft animal model. These results suggest that phomaketide A may impair lymphangiogenesis by suppressing VEGFR-3, PKCδ, and eNOS signaling cascades, while simultaneously activating protease inhibitors in human LECs. We document for the first time that phomaketide A inhibits lymphangiogenesis both *in vitro* and *in vivo*, which suggests that this natural product could potentially treat cancer metastasis.

Keywords: phomaketide A; lymphangiogenesis; lymphatic endothelial cells; vascular endothelial growth factor receptor-3

---

1. Introduction

Cancer metastasis enables cancer cells to spread from the primary tumor and establish themselves in other tissues. Lymphatic circulation is a common route for cancer metastasis [1], with the thin walls and few tight junctions in the lymphatic vessels offering good permeability. Moreover, the lack of basal lamina and associated pericytes, means that lymphatic capillaries have an easy opening for the uptake of macromolecular cancer cells into the lymphatic vessels [2,3]. Lymphangiogenesis, the process by which new lymphatic vessels grow out of pre-existing vessels, enables lymphatic endothelial cells (LECs) to proliferate and migrate through lymphatic vessels surrounding the tumors [4,5]. Lymphangiogenic factors, including vascular endothelial growth factor (VEGF)-C or D, predominantly bind to VEGF receptor-3 (VEGFR-3), and promote several downstream signaling pathways for regulating lymphangiogenesis [6–8]. During the lymphangiogenic process, LEC survival, proliferation, migration and tube formation depends upon the activation of the VEGF-C/VEGFR-3 axis [9]. In various experimental tumor models, overexpression of VEGF-C can induce lymphangiogenesis and disseminate metastatic tumor cells to lymph nodes [10], and the use of neutralizing antibodies against VEGF-C and VEGFR-3 can prevent tumor lymphangiogenesis and lymphatic metastasis [11]. Thus, selective targeting of VEGFR-3-dependent lymphangiogenesis can potentially block cancer progression and metastasis.

Marine bacteria, microalgae and fungi have proven to be a rich source of bioactive metabolites possessing biological and pharmacological properties with enormous therapeutic potential [12]. We have previously demonstrated that phomaketide A, isolated from the marine endophytic fungal strain *Phoma* sp. NTOU4195, exerts anti-angiogenic and anti-inflammatory effects [13]. However, no data exist as to the effects of phomaketide A on tumor lymphangiogenesis. We therefore explored the *in vitro* and *in vivo* anti-lymphangiogenic effects and mechanisms of phomaketide A.

2. Results

2.1. Anti-Lymphangiogeneic Effects of Phomaketide A on Human LECs

To examine the growth-inhibitory effects of phomaketide A (Figure 1A), we treated human LECs with various concentrations of phomaketide A. Figure 1B illustrates how phomaketide A inhibited LECs growth in a concentration-dependent manner (IC_{50} = 3.7 ± 0.6 μM). The lymphangiogenesis inhibitor, rapamycin, served as a positive control [14]. Next, the results of a tube formation assay showed that phomaketide A significantly reduced LECs tube formation (Figure 2A). Since the migratory ability of endothelial cells is another essential characteristic of lymphangiogenesis [15], we therefore evaluated the effect of phomaketide A on LECs migration. We found that phomaketide A markedly reduced the numbers of LECs that migrated through the Transwell inserts (Figure 2B).

Moreover, there were no discernable increase on the levels of lactate dehydrogenase (LDH) with either dose of phomaketide A as compared with untreated human LECs (controls) (Figure 2D). Thus, phomaketide A appears to exert anti-lymphangiogenic effects without any evidence of cytotoxicity in human LECs.

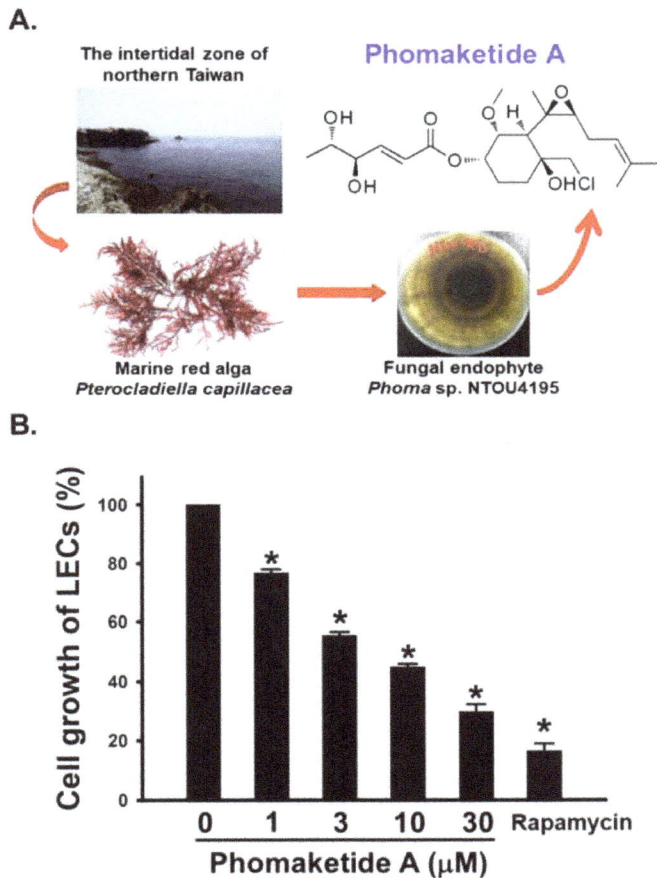

Figure 1. Effects of phomaketide A on cell growth of human lymphatic endothelial cells (LECs). (**A**) Phomaketide A was identified from the fermented broth and mycelium of *Phoma* sp. NTOU4195 isolated from the marine red alga *Pterocladiella capillacea* harvested along the north coast of Taiwan. (**B**) Cells were treated with various concentrations of phomaketide A and rapamycin (10 μM) for 48 h, and anti-lymphangiogenic activity was explored in a cell growth assay (N = 3). Data are expressed as the mean ± SEM. * $p < 0.05$ compared with the control group.

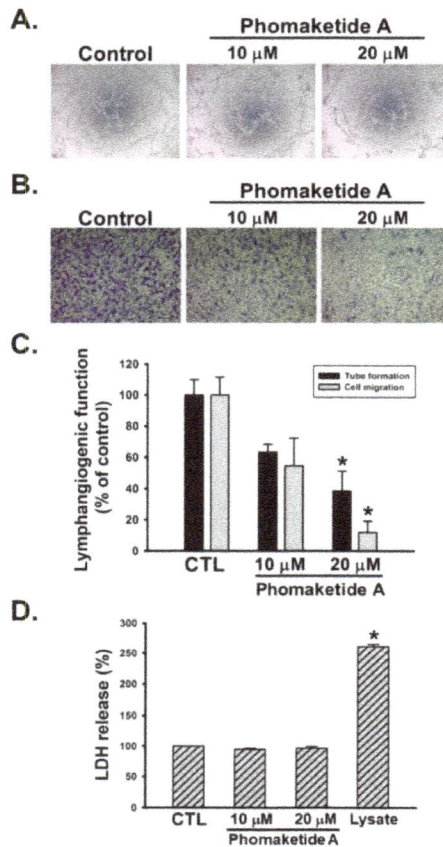

Figure 2. Effects of phomaketide A on human LECs tube formation, migration, and cytotoxicity. Cells were treated with the indicated concentrations of phomaketide A for 8 h. Capillary-like structure formation (**A**) and cell migration (**B**) were examined by tube formation and Transwell assays, respectively (N = 4–6). (**C**) ImageJ software was used to validate the lymphangiogenic functions of phomaketide A. (**D**) Cells were treated with phomaketide A for 24 h, then cytotoxicity was evaluated by lactate dehydrogenase (LDH) assay (N = 3). Data are expressed as the mean ± SEM. * $p < 0.05$ compared with the control (CTL) group.

2.2. Phomaketide A Inhibits the VEGFR-3 and PKCδ Signaling Pathway in Human LECs

To elucidate the mechanisms employed by phomaketide A to regulate lymphangiogenesis, we explored its effects upon VEGFR-3 in LECs. Figure 3A,B illustrate the significant suppression by phomaketide A upon the phosphorylation of VEGFR-3. We also investigated the effects of phomaketide A upon the signal transduction downstream of VEGFR-3. The results indicated that phomaketide A dramatically decreased the phosphorylation of PKCδ, but did not affect the phosphorylated levels of Akt, Erk, or FAK in the LECs (Figure 3C,D). Our results demonstrate that phomaketide A reduces lymphangiogenesis through VEGFR-3 and PKCδ-dependent pathways in human LECs.

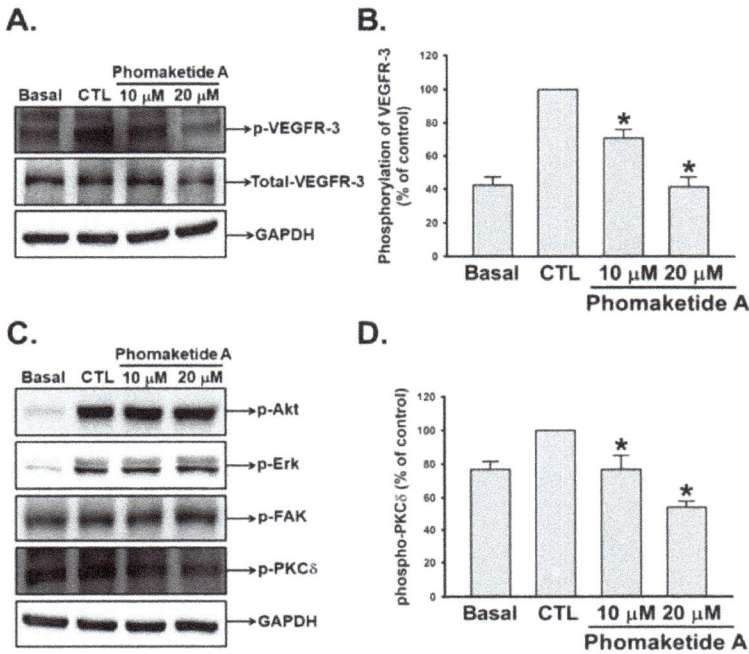

Figure 3. Modulation of phomaketide A on VEGFR-3 and downstream signaling pathways in human LECs. (**A** and **C**) Quiescent LECs were treated with or without EGM-2MV medium in the absence (CTL) or presence of phomaketide A for 5–10 min. The phosphorylation of VEGFR-3, Akt, Erk, FAK, and PKCδ were determined by Western blot analysis (N = 5–7). The quantitative densitometry of the relative levels of phosphorylated VEGFR-3 and PKCδ were measured by Image-Pro Plus processing software (**B** and **D**). Data are expressed as the mean ± SEM. * $p < 0.05$ compared with the control (CTL) group.

2.3. Phomaketide A Impedes eNOS Activation in Human LECs

Recent studies have documented that integrin α9, integrin β1, and endothelial nitric oxide synthase (eNOS) were associated with VEGFR-3-mediated lymphangiogenesis [8,16,17]. We therefore investigated whether phomaketide A inhibits LECs-induced lymphangiogenesis via these molecular signals. We found that phomaketide A significantly suppressed the phosphorylation and expression of eNOS but did not impair the protein levels of integrin α9 and β1 (Figure 4A,B). Activation of nuclear factor-κB (NF-κB) and overexpression of Id-1 (inhibitor of differentiation/DNA binding) are critical for multiple physiological and pathological processes, including lymphangiogenesis [17–19]. Here, we found that phomaketide A did not alter the phosphorylation of p65 or IκBα, nor the expression of Id-1 in LECs. We suggest that the eNOS signaling pathway is involved in phomaketide A-induced anti-lymphangiogenic effects in human LECs.

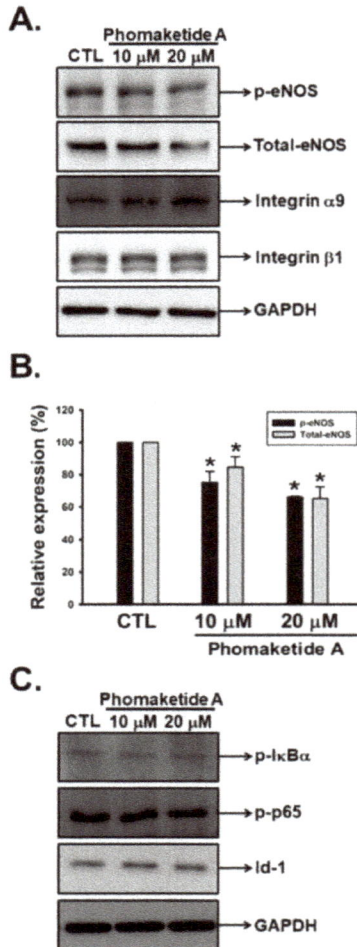

Figure 4. Effects of phomaketide A on pro-lymphangiogenic signals and transcription factors in human LECs. (**A** and **C**) Cells were treated with the indicated concentrations of phomaketide A for 8 h, and the indicated phosphorylated and total proteins were determined by Western blot analysis (N = 4–6). Image-Pro Plus processing software quantified the relative level of protein (**B**). Data are expressed as the mean ± SEM. * $p < 0.05$ compared with the control (CTL) group.

2.4. Phomaketide A Increases the Expression Profile of Protease Inhibitors in Human LECs

Proteolytic activities of cells are coordinately regulated by proteases and protease inhibitors in a coordinated fashion for the degradation of the extracellular matrix (ECM). Analysis of protease and/or protease inhibitor expression profiles is essential to determine how they affect normal cellular function and dysregulate LECs lymphangiogenesis [20]. Using human proteome arrays, we found that phomaketide A did not affect the relative expression of 35 human proteases (Supplementary Figure 1). However, phomaketide A substantially increased the levels of protein expression of several human protease inhibitors in LECs (Figure 5A); the four most significantly upregulated protease inhibitors were cystatin A, serpin B6, tissue factor pathway inhibitor (TFPI), and tissue inhibitor matrix metalloproteinase 1 (TIMP-1) (Figure 5B). These results indicate that phomaketide A may inhibit lymphangiogenesis via the upregulation of cystatin A, serpin B6, TFPI, and TIMP-1 in LECs.

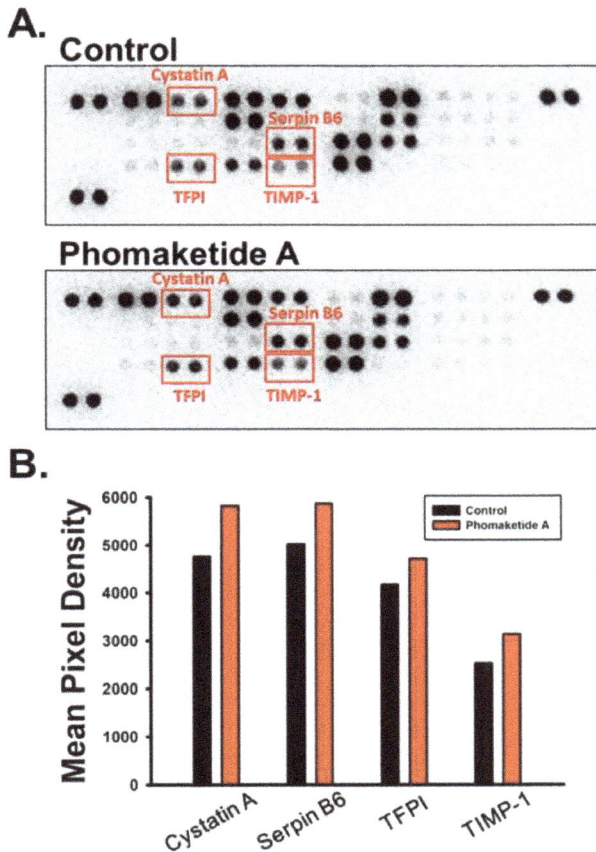

Figure 5. Effects of phomaketide A on protease inhibitor expression profiles in human LECs. (**A**) LECs were treated with phomaketide A (20 μM) for 8 h, then total cell lysates were collected. Significant changes in protein spots detected by human protease inhibitor array are indicated. (**B**) Profiles of mean spot pixel densities for upregulated protease inhibitors were analyzed using ImageJ software.

2.5. Phomaketide A Impairs Tumor Lymphangiogenesis in the A549 Xenograft Model

To validate *in vivo* significance of the cellular observations, we determined the effect of phomaketide A on tumor xenograft growth. As shown in Figure 6A, phomaketide A repressed A549 tumor growth via a remarkable reduction of bioluminescence activity. Furthermore, we found that phomaketide A dramatically decreased the tumor volume and weight of A549 xenografts (Figure 6B,C). Immunohistochemical analysis revealed that the expression of LYVE-1, the key specific marker for lymphatic vessels [21], was obviously decreased by phomaketide A (Figure 6D). Based on these findings, we propose that phomaketide A blocks *in vivo* tumor progression by suppressing lymphangiogenesis.

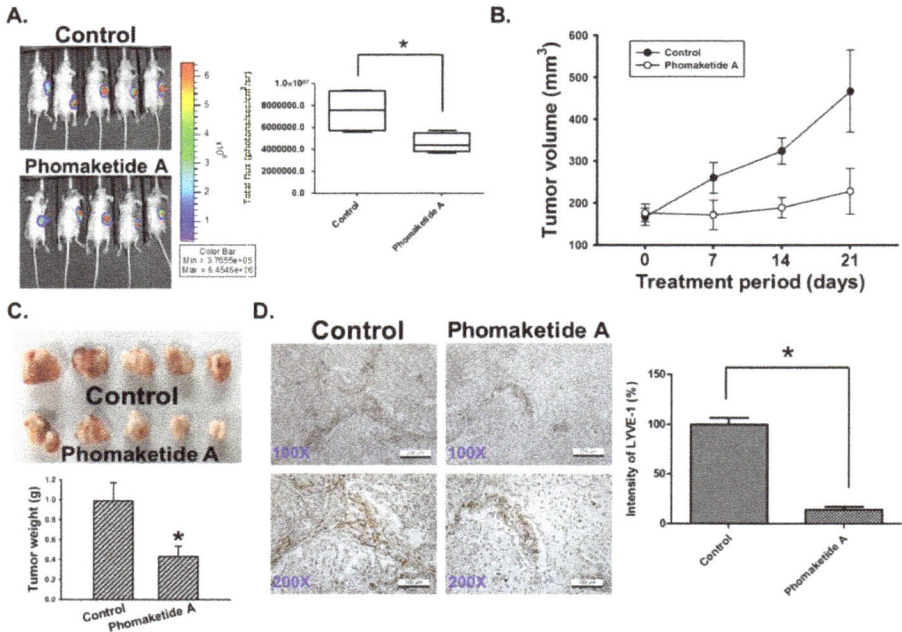

Figure 6. Effects of phomaketide A on tumor-associated lymphangiogenesis. (**A**) A549-Leu cells were injected into flank sites of nude mice for 4 weeks. Then, animals (five mice/group) were given vehicle (control) and phomaketide A (20 mg/kg) by i.p. injection for 3 consecutive weeks. The tumor size was monitored by bioluminescence imaging. Representative IVIS images of tumor growth and quantitative analysis of imaging signal intensity was seen on day 21. (**B**) Treatment period was indicated (days 0–21), and tumor volume was measured manually every week. (**C**) A549 tumor samples from animals were obtained and weighted at the end of the treatment. (**D**) The xenograft tumors were excised and stained with lymphatic vessel marker LYVE-1 by IHC analysis (N = 4). Representative images of LYVE-1 expression in tumor specimens are seen. The quantification of LYVE-1 expression was analyzed using ImageJ software. Data are expressed as the mean ± SEM. *, $p < 0.05$ compared with the control group.

3. Discussion

Several studies have shown that marine-derived compounds possess biological activity and pharmacological effect in cancer models with little or no side effects [22–24]. To our knowledge, this is the first study illustrating the anti-lymphangiogenesis property of phomaketide A. Marine organisms are the cradle for many excellent pharmaceutical products, particularly in anti-lymphangiogenesis. For example, fucoidan from *Undaria pinnatifida* sporophylls exerts anti-metastasis and anti-lymphangiogenesis activities by reducing HIF-1α/VEGF-C resulting in attenuation of the PI3K/Akt/mTOR signaling pathways [25]. In addition, toluquinol, isolated from the culture broth of the marine fungus *Penicillium* sp. HL-85-ALS5-R004, has been reported to suppress lymphangiogenesis by down-regulating the VEGF-C/VEGFR-3 cascade [26]. A recent study has shown that tuberazines C obtained from Taiwanese zoanthid *Palythoa tuberculosa* displayed the anti-lymphangiogenesis effect through the suppression of cell growth and tube formation in human LECs [14]. Here, we discover that phomaketide A, isolated from the marine endophytic fungal strain *Phoma* sp. NTOU4195 [13], possesses the anti-lymphangiogenic function against human LECs. Marine-derived natural product phomaketide A has the potential to impede tumor-associated lymphangiogenesis and metastasis.

VEGFR-3 has been reported to play an important role in lymphangiogenesis and tumor invasion through the lymphatics [27]. On stimulation by its ligand VEGF-C, VEGFR-3 was phosphorylated which promotes the proliferation and migration of LECs resulting in lymphangiogenesis [9]. Previous studies showed that Ki23057 inhibits phosphorylation of VEGFR-3 against the lymphangiogenesis of gastric cancer [27]. In the current study, we demonstrated that phomaketide A significantly inhibited the phosphorylation of VEGFR-3 in human LECs. Moreover, PKC δ is associated with the phosphorylation of VEGFR-3 in endothelial cells [28]. Our results found that phomaketide A also induced the reduction of PKCδ phosphorylation. PKCδ mediated by VEGFR-3 phosphorylation underlying phomaketide A treatment deserves further investigation. In addition, eNOS is involved in VEGF-C-induced lymphangiogenesis and plays a vital role in lymphatic metastasis [8]. Doxycycline can decrease eNOS phosphorylation to inhibit LECs proliferation [29]. Pro-inflammatory cytokines, IL-20 and IL-33, also activate the phosphorylation of eNOS to promote the proliferation, migration and tube formation of LECs [30,31]. In the current study, phomaketide A suppressed the phosphorylation and expression of eNOS in LECs, confirming the importance of eNOS in LECs-regulated lymphangiogenic processes.

Proteolytic processing of VEGF-C regulates lymphatic vessel growth for activating LECs lymphangiogenesis [32,33], whereas lymphatic vessel outgrowth is reduced by protease inhibitor [34]. Several studies demonstrate that serine proteinase inhibitor (serpin) functioned as a lymphangiogenesis inhibitor to suppress the lymphatic metastasis of cancer and the LECs proliferation and migration [35–37]. The expression of tissue inhibitor of metalloproteinase-2 (TIMP-2) is lower or negative in patients with lymph node metastasis [38]. Furthermore, matrix metalloproteinases inhibitors are well recognized to impair lymphangiogenesis [39]. Our results showed that anti-lymphangiogenic effects of phomaketide A were associated with the induction of protease inhibitors such as cystatin A, serpin B6, TFPI and TIMP-1. Meanwhile, several studies have demonstrated that promotion of these protease inhibitors can induce anti-angiogenic effects [40–43]. Our previous report reveals that phomaketide A is a novel angiogenesis inhibitor [13]. Phomaketide A is a potential dual-effect agent that could be used for cancer treatment through the inhibition of angiogenesis and lymphangiogenesis.

In conclusion, this report discloses a novel mechanism by which phomaketide A reduces LECs lymphangiogenesis *in vitro* and *in vivo*. We demonstrate that phomaketide A antagonizes lymphangiogenesis by decreasing VEGFR-3 and its downstream PKCδ and eNOS signaling pathways, as well as increasing protease inhibitors in human LECs (Figure 7). Our previous study demonstrates promising *in vitro* effects with phomaketide A in human EPCs. In this study, we show that phomaketide A also exerts anti-lymphangiogenic effect in LECs (IC$_{50}$, 3.7 $\pm$ 0.6 μM), and profoundly inhibit the proliferation of A549 lung cancer cells, with an IC$_{50}$ value of 3.0 $\pm$ 0.3 μM (Supplementary Figure S2). We therefore suggest that phomaketide A acts selective and potent inhibitory effects upon endothelial cells and A549 cancer cells. Phomaketide A can coordinately induce anti-angiogenic, anti-lymphangiogenic, and anti-cancer effects in A549 tumor microenvironment, resulting in the inhibition of *in vivo* tumor progression. The detailed anti-cancer effects and mechanisms of phomaketide A in A549 cancer cells should be further investigated. LECs have been proposed to dictate tumor lymphangiogenesis and metastasis in microenvironment. Our findings suggest that phomaketide A may serve as a lead candidate for further development for novel lymphangiogenesis inhibitors to block cancer progression and metastasis.

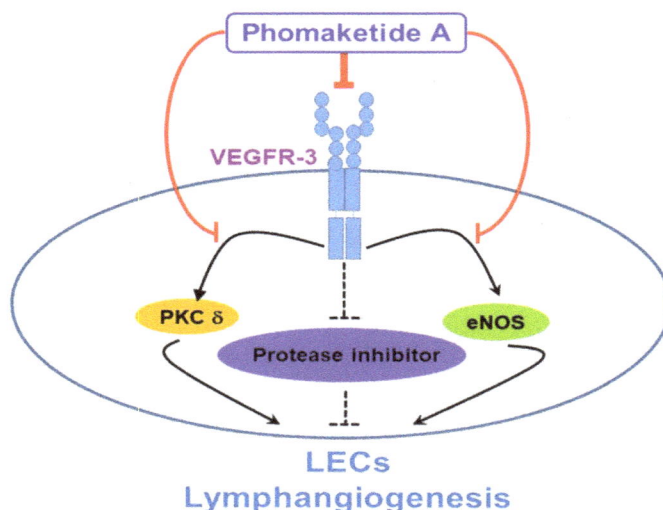

Figure 7. Schema of phomaketide A-induced anti-lymphangiogenic mechanism in human LECs. This study reveals phomaketide A as a promising anti-lymphangiogenic agent. Phomaketide A may inhibit lymphangiogenesis by decreasing VEGFR-3 and its downstream PKCδ and eNOS signaling pathways, as well as increasing protease inhibitors in human LECs.

4. Materials and Methods

4.1. Materials

Phomaketide A was isolated from the fermentation broth and mycelium of the endophytic fungal strain *Phoma* sp. NTOU4195 as previously described [13]. Rapamycin was purchased from Cayman Chemical (Ann Arbor, MI, USA). The compounds were dissolved in dimethyl sulfoxide (DMSO) at 20 mM as a stock solution for all assays. DMSO was used as the vehicle control in the experiments. DMSO and other chemical agents were obtained from Sigma-Aldrich (St. Louis, MO, USA). Rabbit polyclonal antibody specific for phospho-VEGFR-3 (Tyr1230/1231) was purchased from Cell Application (San Diego, CA, USA). Rabbit monoclonal antibodies specific for phospho-Akt (Ser473), phospho-ERK (Thr202/Tyr204), phospho-FAK (Tyr397), phospho-PKCδ (Thr505), phospho-eNOS (Ser1177), eNOS, Integrin β1, VEGFR-3, and GAPDH were purchased from Cell Signaling Technologies (Boston, MA, USA). Rabbit monoclonal antibodies specific for Integrin α9, phospho-p65 (Ser536) and phospho-IκBα (Ser32) were purchased from Abcam (Cambridge, MA, USA). Rabbit polyclonal antibody specific for Id-1 was purchased from Santa Cruz Biotechnology (Santa Cruz, CA, USA). Gibco-BRL life technologies (Grand Island, NY, USA) supplied Dulbecco's modified Eagle's medium (DMEM), fetal bovine serum (FBS), and all other cell culture reagents. Matrigel was obtained from BD Biosciences (Bedford, MA, USA).

4.2. Cell Culture

The human lymphatic endothelial cells (LECs) were purchased from Lonza (Walkersville, MD, USA). LECs were cultured in EGM-2MV medium consisting of EBM-2 basal medium and SingleQuots kit (Lonza). A549 cell line was purchased from American Type Culture Collection (Manassas, Virginia, USA). To establish the luciferase-tagged A549 cells (A549-Leu cells), pLenti PGK Blast V5-LUC (w528-1) for expression of the firefly luciferase was purchased from the Addgene (Plasmid #19166; Watertown, MA, USA). Lentiviruses were prepared according to standard protocols. For transduction, 3×10^5 A549 cells were seeded in a 6-well plate and the lentivirus was added (multiplicity of infection =

10) in medium containing polybrene (8 μg/mL). The culture medium was changed after 24 h. The cells were incubated with 5 μg/mL blasticidin for 48 h for stable clone selection. The surviving cells were selected, and clonal cell populations were expanded as A549-Luc cell line. A549-Leu cells were maintained in DMEM, supplemented with 10% fetal bovine serum (FBS). The cells culture conditions are recorded in our previous paper [14].

4.3. Cell Growth Assay

LECs were cultured in 96-well plates at a density of 5×10^3 cells in each well. Overnight, the culture medium was replaced with fresh EGM-2MV medium in the presence of either vehicle (DMSO) or phomaketide A for 48 h treatment. The assay on cell growth of LECs was determined by the method based on our previous study [14].

4.4. Capillary Tube Formation Assay

The capillary tube formation assay was performed on Matrigel-coated 96-well plates. LECs were seeded at a density of 2×10^4 cells per well and incubated in EGM-2MV medium and the indicated concentration of tested compounds, for 8 h at 37 °C. The detection and quantification of LECs tube formation were examined according to previously described procedures [14].

4.5. Cell Migration Assay

The cell migration assay was conducted in Transwell inserts (Corning, NY, USA) with 2.5×10^4 of LECs per well seeded onto the upper chamber with EBM-2 basal medium. The upper chamber was transferred and incubated in the bottom chamber with EGM-2MV medium and the indicated concentration of tested compounds was for 8 h. Cell migration was determined according to our previous protocol [44].

4.6. Cytotoxicity Assay

LECs (5×10^3 cells/well) were seeded onto 96-well plates and incubated with EGM-2MV medium in the presence of a vehicle (DMSO) or phomaketide A for 8 h of treatment. Release of lactate dehydrogenase (LDH) into the medium was measured using a cytotoxicity assay kit (Promega, Madison, WI, USA) according to an established protocol [14].

4.7. Western Blot Analysis

After the treatment of LECs, the reaction was terminated by the addition of lysis buffer containing a protease inhibitor cocktail (Roche, Mannheim, Germany). Total cell lysates were electrophoresed using SDS-PAGE and subsequently transferred to polyvinylidene difluoride membranes. After blocking the blots with 4% bovine serum albumin, they were treated with primary antibody and then peroxidase-conjugated secondary antibody. The blots were visualized using enhanced chemiluminescence and monitored using the UVP Biospectrum system (UVP, Upland, CA, USA).

4.8. Proteome Profile Arrays

Human protease and protease inhibitor antibody arrays (R&D Systems, Minneapolis, MN, USA) were used to analyze the expression profiles of protease and protease inhibitor according to the manufacturer's instructions. UVP Biospectrum system was used to detect chemiluminescent signals, which were further analyzed using ImageJ software.

4.9. In Vivo Tumor Xenograft Model

All animal procedures were performed according to approved protocols issued by the China Medical University (Taichung, Taiwan) Institutional Animal Care and Use Committees. Male nude mice (4-week of age) were used in the subcutaneous xenograft model. A549-Leu cells (2×10^6 cells) were resuspended in 0.1 mL of 50% serum-free medium and 50% Matrigel, and injected into the right flank of each animal. Four weeks after A549-Leu cells injection, the mice were randomized into experimental and control groups according to bioluminescence imaging from the Xenogen IVIS imaging system 200 (PerkinElmer, MA, USA). Then, the mice were treated with phomaketide A (20 mg/kg) or the vehicle control every other day by intraperitoneal (i.p.) administration (five mice per group). After the treatment, the animals were sacrificed, and the tumor specimens were resected for immunohistochemical (IHC) analysis.

4.10. IHC Analysis

The tumor tissues were placed on glass slides, rehydrated and incubated in 3% hydrogen peroxide to block the endogenous peroxidase activity. After trypsinization, nonspecific antibody-binding sites were blocked using 3% bovine serum albumin in PBS. IHC analysis was carried out to determine the expression of lymphangiogenic marker according to the standard protocol [45].

4.11. Statistical Analysis

Data points represent the mean ± standard error of mean (SEM). Statistical analyses of data were done with one-way ANOVA followed by Student's t-test. The difference is significant if the *p* value is < 0.05.

Supplementary Materials: The following are available online at http://www.mdpi.com/1660-3397/17/4/215/s1, Figure S1: Effect of phomaketide A on the expression profile of proteases in human LECs. Figure S2: Effect of phomaketide A on cell growth of A549 cancer cells.

Author Contributions: S.-W.W., C.-H.T., and Y.-J.C. designed and conceived the study. T.-H.L. and M.-S.L. isolated and purified the phomaketide A. H.-C.T., L.-P.C., P.-C.C. and C.-Y.L. performed the experimental work and drew the diagrams. C.-W.C., C.-T.L., and S.-S.C. analyzed and interpreted the data. H.-C.T., K.-W.L., C.-H.L. and S.-W.W. wrote and revised the manuscript, W.-C.C. validated the manuscript. All authors read and approved the final manuscript.

Funding: This research was funded by (Ministry of Science and Technology, Taiwan) grant number (MOST 106-2320-B-715-001-MY3; MOST 107-2320-B-030-005), (Mackay Medical College) grant number (MMC-1071B27), (MacKay Memorial Hospital) grant number (MMH-108-94), and (Taipei City Hospital) grant number (TCH 10701-62-027). The APC was funded by Mackay Medical College.

Acknowledgments: We thank Iona J. MacDonald for her English language editing of this manuscript.

Conflicts of Interest: The authors declare no conflicts of interest.

References

1. Paduch, R. The role of lymphangiogenesis and angiogenesis in tumor metastasis. *Cell. Oncol. (Dordr.)* **2016**, *39*, 397–410. [CrossRef] [PubMed]

2. Tammela, T.; Alitalo, K. Lymphangiogenesis: Molecular mechanisms and future promise. *Cell* **2010**, *140*, 460–476. [CrossRef] [PubMed]

3. Alderfer, L.; Wei, A.; Hanjaya-Putra, D. Lymphatic Tissue Engineering and Regeneration. *J. Biol. Eng.* **2018**, *12*, 32. [CrossRef] [PubMed]

4. Kataru, R.P.; Kim, H.; Jang, C.; Choi, D.K.; Koh, B.I.; Kim, M.; Gollamudi, S.; Kim, Y.K.; Lee, S.H.; Koh, G.Y. T lymphocytes negatively regulate lymph node lymphatic vessel formation. *Immunity* **2011**, *34*, 96–107. [CrossRef]

5. Yeo, K.P.; Angeli, V. Bidirectional Crosstalk between Lymphatic Endothelial Cell and T Cell and Its Implications in Tumor Immunity. *Front. Immunol.* **2017**, *8*, 83. [CrossRef]

6. Stacker, S.A.; Williams, S.P.; Karnezis, T.; Shayan, R.; Fox, S.B.; Achen, M.G. Lymphangiogenesis and lymphatic vessel remodelling in cancer. *Nat. Rev. Cancer* **2014**, *14*, 159–172. [CrossRef] [PubMed]

7. Vaahtomeri, K.; Karaman, S.; Makinen, T.; Alitalo, K. Lymphangiogenesis guidance by paracrine and pericellular factors. *Genes Dev.* **2017**, *31*, 1615–1634. [CrossRef]

8. Lahdenranta, J.; Hagendoorn, J.; Padera, T.P.; Hoshida, T.; Nelson, G.; Kashiwagi, S.; Jain, R.K.; Fukumura, D. Endothelial nitric oxide synthase mediates lymphangiogenesis and lymphatic metastasis. *Cancer Res.* **2009**, *69*, 2801–2808. [CrossRef] [PubMed]

9. Makinen, T.; Veikkola, T.; Mustjoki, S.; Karpanen, T.; Catimel, B.; Nice, E.C.; Wise, L.; Mercer, A.; Kowalski, H.; Kerjaschki, D.; et al. Isolated lymphatic endothelial cells transduce growth, survival and migratory signals via the VEGF-C/D receptor VEGFR-3. *EMBO J.* **2001**, *20*, 4762–4773. [CrossRef] [PubMed]

10. Alam, A.; Blanc, I.; Gueguen-Dorbes, G.; Duclos, O.; Bonnin, J.; Barron, P.; Laplace, M.C.; Morin, G.; Gaujarengues, F.; Dol, F.; et al. SAR131675, a potent and selective VEGFR-3-TK inhibitor with antilymphangiogenic, antitumoral, and antimetastatic activities. *Mol. Cancer Ther.* **2012**, *11*, 1637–1649. [CrossRef] [PubMed]

11. Norrmen, C.; Tammela, T.; Petrova, T.V.; Alitalo, K. Biological basis of therapeutic lymphangiogenesis. *Circulation* **2011**, *123*, 1335–1351. [CrossRef]

12. Rateb, M.E.; Ebel, R. Secondary metabolites of fungi from marine habitats. *Nat. Prod. Rep.* **2011**, *28*, 290–344. [CrossRef] [PubMed]

13. Lee, M.S.; Wang, S.W.; Wang, G.J.; Pang, K.L.; Lee, C.K.; Kuo, Y.H.; Cha, H.J.; Lin, R.K.; Lee, T.H. Angiogenesis Inhibitors and Anti-Inflammatory Agents from Phoma sp. NTOU4195. *J. Nat. Prod.* **2016**, *79*, 2983–2990. [CrossRef] [PubMed]

14. Chen, S.R.; Wang, S.W.; Su, C.J.; Hu, H.C.; Yang, Y.L.; Hsieh, C.T.; Peng, C.C.; Chang, F.R.; Cheng, Y.B. Anti-Lymphangiogenesis Components from Zoanthid Palythoa tuberculosa. *Mar. Drugs* **2018**, *16*, 47. [CrossRef] [PubMed]

15. Prangsaengtong, O.; Athikomkulchai, S.; Xu, J.; Koizumi, K.; Inujima, A.; Shibahara, N.; Shimada, Y.; Tadtong, S.; Awale, S. Chrysin Inhibits Lymphangiogenesis in Vitro. *Biol. Pharm. Bull.* **2016**, *39*, 466–472. [CrossRef]

16. Urner, S.; Planas-Paz, L.; Hilger, L.S.; Henning, C.; Branopolski, A.; Kelly-Goss, M.; Stanczuk, L.; Pitter, B.; Montanez, E.; Peirce, S.M.; et al. Identification of ILK as a critical regulator of VEGFR3 signalling and lymphatic vascular growth. *EMBO J.* **2019**, *38*, e99322. [CrossRef]

17. Flister, M.J.; Wilber, A.; Hall, K.L.; Iwata, C.; Miyazono, K.; Nisato, R.E.; Pepper, M.S.; Zawieja, D.C.; Ran, S. Inflammation induces lymphangiogenesis through up-regulation of VEGFR-3 mediated by NF-kappaB and Prox1. *Blood* **2010**, *115*, 418–429. [CrossRef]

18. Dong, Z.; Wei, F.; Zhou, C.; Sumida, T.; Hamakawa, H.; Hu, Y.; Liu, S. Silencing Id-1 inhibits lymphangiogenesis through down-regulation of VEGF-C in oral squamous cell carcinoma. *Oral Oncol.* **2011**, *47*, 27–32. [CrossRef]

19. Si, C.F.; Guo, J.Q.; Yang, Y.M.; Zhang, N.; Pan, C.R.; Zhang, Q.H.; Zhang, T.G.; Zhou, C.J. Nuclear and cytoplasmic Id-1 expression patterns play different roles in angiogenesis and lymphangiogenesis in gastric carcinoma. *Ann. Diagn. Pathol.* **2011**, *15*, 46–51. [CrossRef]

20. Leppanen, V.M.; Tvorogov, D.; Kisko, K.; Prota, A.E.; Jeltsch, M.; Anisimov, A.; Markovic-Mueller, S.; Stuttfeld, E.; Goldie, K.N.; Ballmer-Hofer, K.; et al. Structural and mechanistic insights into VEGF receptor 3 ligand binding and activation. *Proc. Natl. Acad. Sci. USA* **2013**, *110*, 12960–12965. [CrossRef] [PubMed]

21. Banerji, S.; Ni, J.; Wang, S.X.; Clasper, S.; Su, J.; Tammi, R.; Jones, M.; Jackson, D.G. LYVE-1, a new homologue of the CD44 glycoprotein, is a lymph-specific receptor for hyaluronan. *J. Cell Biol.* **1999**, *144*, 789–801. [CrossRef] [PubMed]

22. Castro-Carvalho, B.; Ramos, A.A.; Prata-Sena, M.; Malhao, F.; Moreira, M.; Gargiulo, D.; Dethoup, T.; Buttachon, S.; Kijjoa, A.; Rocha, E. Marine-derived Fungi Extracts Enhance the Cytotoxic Activity of Doxorubicin in Nonsmall Cell Lung Cancer Cells A459. *Pharmacogn. Res.* **2017**, *9* (Suppl. S1), S92–S98.

23. Aspeslagh, S.; Stein, M.; Bahleda, R.; Hollebecque, A.; Salles, G.; Gyan, E.; Fudio, S.; Extremera, S.; Alfaro, V.; Soto-Matos, A.; et al. Phase I dose-escalation study of plitidepsin in combination with sorafenib or gemcitabine in patients with refractory solid tumors or lymphomas. *Anticancer Drugs* **2017**, *28*, 341–349. [CrossRef] [PubMed]

24. Yu, C.I.; Chen, C.Y.; Liu, W.; Chang, P.C.; Huang, C.W.; Han, K.F.; Lin, I.P.; Lin, M.Y.; Lee, C.H. Sandensolide Induces Oxidative Stress-Mediated Apoptosis in Oral Cancer Cells and in Zebrafish Xenograft Model. *Mar. Drugs* **2018**, *16*, 387. [CrossRef] [PubMed]

25. Teng, H.; Yang, Y.; Wei, H.; Liu, Z.; Liu, Z.; Ma, Y.; Gao, Z.; Hou, L.; Zou, X. Fucoidan Suppresses Hypoxia-Induced Lymphangiogenesis and Lymphatic Metastasis in Mouse Hepatocarcinoma. *Mar. Drugs* **2015**, *13*, 3514–3530. [CrossRef]
26. Garcia-Caballero, M.; Blacher, S.; Paupert, J.; Quesada, A.R.; Medina, M.A.; Noel, A. Novel application assigned to toluquinol: Inhibition of lymphangiogenesis by interfering with VEGF-C/VEGFR-3 signalling pathway. *Br. J. Pharmacol.* **2016**, *173*, 1966–1987. [CrossRef]
27. Yashiro, M.; Shinto, O.; Nakamura, K.; Tendo, M.; Matsuoka, T.; Matsuzaki, T.; Kaizaki, R.; Ohira, M.; Miwa, A.; Hirakawa, K. Effects of VEGFR-3 phosphorylation inhibitor on lymph node metastasis in an orthotopic diffuse-type gastric carcinoma model. *Br. J. Cancer* **2009**, *101*, 1100–1106. [CrossRef]
28. Wang, J.F.; Zhang, X.; Groopman, J.E. Activation of vascular endothelial growth factor receptor-3 and its downstream signaling promote cell survival under oxidative stress. *J. Biol. Chem.* **2004**, *279*, 27088–27097. [CrossRef]
29. Han, L.; Su, W.; Huang, J.; Zhou, J.; Qiu, S.; Liang, D. Doxycycline inhibits inflammation-induced lymphangiogenesis in mouse cornea by multiple mechanisms. *PLoS ONE* **2014**, *9*, e108931. [CrossRef]
30. Han, L.; Zhang, M.; Liang, X.; Jia, X.; Jia, J.; Zhao, M.; Fan, Y. Interleukin-33 promotes inflammation-induced lymphangiogenesis via ST2/TRAF6-mediated Akt/eNOS/NO signalling pathway. *Sci. Rep.* **2017**, *7*, 10602. [CrossRef]
31. Hammer, T.; Tritsaris, K.; Hubschmann, M.V.; Gibson, J.; Nisato, R.E.; Pepper, M.S.; Dissing, S. IL-20 activates human lymphatic endothelial cells causing cell signalling and tube formation. *Microvasc. Res.* **2009**, *78*, 25–32. [CrossRef]
32. Jeltsch, M.; Jha, S.K.; Tvorogov, D.; Anisimov, A.; Leppanen, V.M.; Holopainen, T.; Kivela, R.; Ortega, S.; Karpanen, T.; Alitalo, K. CCBE1 enhances lymphangiogenesis via A disintegrin and metalloprotease with thrombospondin motifs-3-mediated vascular endothelial growth factor-C activation. *Circulation* **2014**, *129*, 1962–1971. [CrossRef]
33. Bui, H.M.; Enis, D.; Robciuc, M.R.; Nurmi, H.J.; Cohen, J.; Chen, M.; Yang, Y.; Dhillon, V.; Johnson, K.; Zhang, H.; et al. Proteolytic activation defines distinct lymphangiogenic mechanisms for VEGFC and VEGFD. *J. Clin. Investig.* **2016**, *126*, 2167–2180. [CrossRef]
34. Detry, B.; Bruyere, F.; Erpicum, C.; Paupert, J.; Lamaye, F.; Maillard, C.; Lenoir, B.; Foidart, J.M.; Thiry, M.; Noel, A. Digging deeper into lymphatic vessel formation in vitro and in vivo. *BMC Cell Biol.* **2011**, *12*, 29. [CrossRef]
35. Ma, C.; Luo, C.; Yin, H.; Zhang, Y.; Xiong, W.; Zhang, T.; Gao, T.; Wang, X.; Che, D.; Fang, Z.; et al. Kallistatin inhibits lymphangiogenesis and lymphatic metastasis of gastric cancer by downregulating VEGF-C expression and secretion. *Gastric Cancer* **2018**, *21*, 617–631. [CrossRef] [PubMed]
36. Ma, C.; Yin, H.; Zhong, J.; Zhang, Y.; Luo, C.; Che, D.; Fang, Z.; Li, L.; Qin, S.; Liang, J.; et al. Kallistatin exerts anti-lymphangiogenic effects by inhibiting lymphatic endothelial cell proliferation, migration and tube formation. *Int. J. Oncol.* **2017**, *50*, 2000–2010. [CrossRef] [PubMed]
37. Liu, Z.; Shi, Y.; Meng, W.; Liu, Y.; Yang, K.; Wu, S.; Peng, Z. Expression and localization of maspin in cervical cancer and its role in tumor progression and lymphangiogenesis. *Arch. Gynecol. Obstet.* **2014**, *289*, 373–382. [CrossRef]
38. Yang, X.; Zhai, N.; Sun, M.; Zhao, Z.; Yang, J.; Chen, K.; Zhang, H. Influence of lymphatic endothelial cells on proliferation and invasiveness of esophageal carcinoma cells in vitro and lymphangiogenesis in vivo. *Med. Oncol.* **2015**, *32*, 222. [CrossRef]
39. Bruyere, F.; Melen-Lamalle, L.; Blacher, S.; Roland, G.; Thiry, M.; Moons, L.; Frankenne, F.; Carmeliet, P.; Alitalo, K.; Libert, C.; et al. Modeling lymphangiogenesis in a three-dimensional culture system. *Nat. Methods* **2008**, *5*, 431–437. [CrossRef]
40. Li, W.; Ding, F.; Zhang, L.; Liu, Z.; Wu, Y.; Luo, A.; Wu, M.; Wang, M.; Zhan, Q.; Liu, Z. Overexpression of stefin A in human esophageal squamous cell carcinoma cells inhibits tumor cell growth, angiogenesis, invasion, and metastasis. *Clin. Cancer Res.* **2005**, *11*, 8753–8762. [CrossRef]
41. Benarafa, C.; Remold-O'Donnell, E. The ovalbumin serpins revisited: Perspective from the chicken genome of clade B serpin evolution in vertebrates. *Proc. Natl. Acad. Sci. USA* **2005**, *102*, 11367–11372. [CrossRef]
42. Zhai, L.L.; Wu, Y.; Huang, D.W.; Tang, Z.G. Increased matrix metalloproteinase-2 expression and reduced tissue factor pathway inhibitor-2 expression correlate with angiogenesis and early postoperative recurrence of pancreatic carcinoma. *Am. J. Transl. Res.* **2015**, *7*, 2412–2422.

43. Abraham, V.; Cao, G.; Parambath, A.; Lawal, F.; Handumrongkul, C.; Debs, R.; DeLisser, H.M. Involvement of TIMP-1 in PECAM-1-mediated tumor dissemination. *Int. J. Oncol.* **2018**, *53*, 488–502. [CrossRef]

44. Chen, W.C.; Chung, C.H.; Lu, Y.C.; Wu, M.H.; Chou, P.H.; Yen, J.Y.; Lai, Y.W.; Wang, G.S.; Liu, S.C.; Cheng, J.K.; et al. BMP-2 induces angiogenesis by provoking integrin alpha6 expression in human endothelial progenitor cells. *Biochem. Pharmacol.* **2018**, *150*, 256–266. [CrossRef]

45. Su, C.M.; Tang, C.H.; Chi, M.J.; Lin, C.Y.; Fong, Y.C.; Liu, Y.C.; Chen, W.C.; Wang, S.W. Resistin facilitates VEGF-C-associated lymphangiogenesis by inhibiting miR-186 in human chondrosarcoma cells. *Biochem. Pharmacol.* **2018**, *154*, 234–242. [CrossRef]

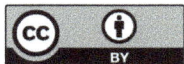

MDPI

St. Alban-Anlage 66

4052 Basel

Switzerland

Tel. +41 61 683 77 34

Fax +41 61 302 89 18

www.mdpi.com

Marine Drugs Editorial Office

E-mail: marinedrugs@mdpi.com

www.mdpi.com/journal/marinedrugs

www.ingramcontent.com/pod-product-compliance
Lightning Source LLC
Chambersburg PA
CBHW051909210326
41597CB00033B/6084